Richard Hoefer, PhD
Editor

Cutting-Edge Social Policy Research

Cutting-Edge Social Policy Research has been co-published simultaneously as *The Social Policy Journal,* Volume 4, Numbers 3/4 2005.

Pre-publication REVIEWS, COMMENTARIES, EVALUATIONS . . .

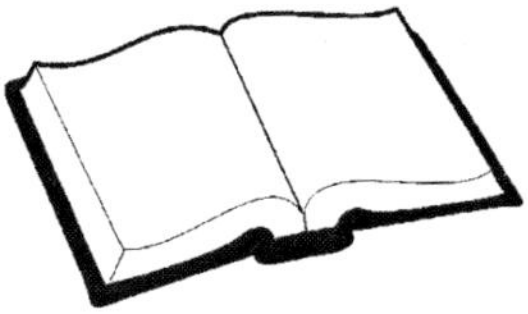

"A VALUABLE READ FOR SOCIAL WORK SCHOLARS AND PRACTITIONERS. Richard Hoefer's craft as an editor is clear in the choice that he makes to include a broad range of contributions that address the needs of at-risk populations, from children who are abused, to adults seeking to maintain their quality of life. He wisely selects multiple research designs that represent best practices in scientific inquiry, including program evaluation, qualitative, and quantitative methodologies."

Deborah Stutevant, PhD
Professor of Theology and Social Work
Hope College

More pre-publication
REVIEWS, COMMENTARIES, EVALUATIONS . . .

"WELL-WRITTEN AND THOUGHTFUL. . . . The book strikes a successful balance between conceptual considerations and concrete suggestions, leaving the reader with plenty to think about and much to do. Particularly helpful are the suggestions regarding methodological changes to make policy findings both more relevant and more readily usable for policymakers."

Sarah-Jane Dodd, PhD
Associate Professor
Hunter College
School of Social Work

"Blending quantitative and qualitative techniques and emphasizing the inclusion of multiple stakeholders in analysis, this book is A WELCOME COMPLEMENT TO STANDARD TEXTBOOKS on policy analysis and development. It provides diverse and sometimes overlooked perspectives on public policy analysis. Two strengths of the book are its emphasis on concretely applying research to policy practice, and its attention to consumers as viable contributors to policy development. The selection of a variety of substantive policy areas to illustrate analytic approaches also should be appealing to policy teachers and students."

Steven G. Anderson, PhD
Associate Professor
School of Social Work
University of Illinois
at Urbana-Champaign

The Haworth Press, Inc.

Cutting-Edge Social Policy Research

Cutting-Edge Social Policy Research has been co-published simultaneously as *The Social Policy Journal*, Volume 4, Numbers 3/4 2005.

Monographic Separates from *The Social Policy Journal*™

For additional information on these and other Haworth Press titles, including descriptions, tables of contents, reviews, and prices, use the QuickSearch catalog at http://www.HaworthPress.com.

Cutting-Edge Social Policy Research, edited by Richard Hoefer, (Vol. 4, No. 3/4, 2005). *"A valuable read for social work scholars and practitioners. Richard Hoefer's craft as an editor is clear in the choice that he makes to include a broad range of contributions that address the needs of at-risk populations, from children who are abused, to adults seeking to maintain their quality of life. He wisely selects multiple research designs that represent best practices in scientific inquiry, including program evaluation, qualitative, and quantitative methodologies." (Deborah Stutevant, PhD, Professor of Theology and Social Work, Hope College)*

Cutting-Edge Social Policy Research

Richard Hoefer, PhD
Editor

Cutting-Edge Social Policy Research has been co-published simultaneously as *The Social Policy Journal*, Volume 4, Numbers 3/4 2005.

The Haworth Press, Inc.

New York • London • Victoria (AU)
www.HaworthPress.com

Cutting-Edge Social Policy Research has been co-published simultaneously as *The Social Policy Journal*, Volume 4, Numbers 3/4 2005.

Cover design by Jennifer M. Gaska

Library of Congress Cataloging-in-Publication Data

Cutting-edge social policy research/Richard Hoefer, editor.
p. cm.
"Cutting-edge social policy research has been co-published simultaneously as The Social policy journal, Vol. 4 numbers 3/4, 2005."
Includes bibliographical references and index.
ISBN-13: 978-0-7890-3205-8 (hard cover. : alk. paper)
ISBN-10: 0-7890-3205-8 (hard cover. : alk. paper)
ISBN-13: 978-0-7890-3206-5 (soft cover. : alk. paper)
ISBN-10: 0-7890-3206-6 (soft cover. : alk. paper)
1. Social policy–Research–Congresses. I. Hoefer, Richard. II Social policy journal.

HN29.C85 2005
361.6′1–dc22

2005030788

Indexing, Abstracting & Website/Internet Coverage

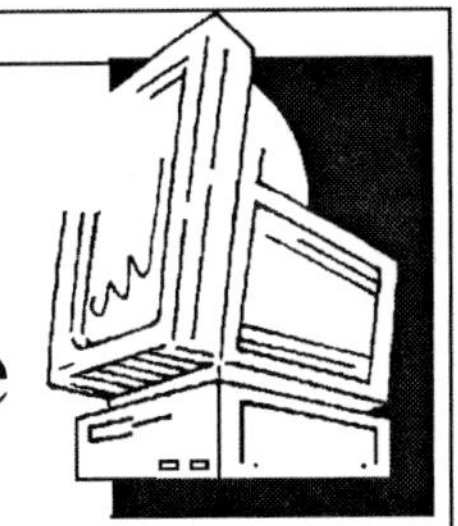

This section provides you with a list of major indexing & abstracting services and other tools for bibliographic access. That is to say, each service began covering this periodical during the year noted in the right column. Most Websites which are listed below have indicated that they will either post, disseminate, compile, archive, cite or alert their own Website users with research-based content from this work. (This list is as current as the copyright date of this publication.)

Abstracting, Website/Indexing Coverage . . . . Year When Coverage Began

- ***CareData: the database supporting social care management and practice <http://www.elsc.org.uk/caredata/caredata.htm>*** . . . **2002**
- ***CINAHL (Cumulative Index to Nursing & Allied Health Literature), in print, EBSCO, and SilverPlatter, DataStar, and PaperChase. (Support materials include Subject Heading List, Database Search Guide, and instructional video) <http://www.cinahl.com>*** . . . **2003**
- ***Criminal Justice Abstracts*** . . . **2003**
- ***DH-Data (available via DataStar and in the HMIC [Health Management Information Consortium] (CD ROM)*** . . . **2003**
- ***Educational Administration Abstracts (EAA)*** . . . **2002**
- ***Elsevier Scopus <http://www.info.scopus.com>*** . . . **2005**
- ***e-psyche, LLC <http://www.e-psyche.net>*** . . . **2002**
- ***Family & Society Studies Worldwide <http://www.nisc.com>*** . . . **2002**
- ***Family Index Database <http://www.familyscholar.com>*** . . . **2003**
- ***Family Violence & Sexual Assault Bulletin*** . . . **2002**
- ***Google <http://www.google.com>*** . . . **2004**

(continued)

- *Google Scholar <http://scholar.google.com>* **2004**
- *Haworth Document Delivery Center <http://www.HaworthPress.com/journals/dds.asp>* **2002**
- *IBZ International Bibliography of Periodical Literature <http://www.saur.de>* **2002**
- *Index to Periodical Articles Related to Law <http://www.law.utexas.edu>* **2002**
- *International Political Science Abstracts. Now also available on CD/ROM and online with data from 1989 to present. Database updated four (4) times a year. Database distributed by EBSCO (cust.serv@epnet.com) and Ovid (sales@ovid.com). <http://www.sciences=po.fr/docum/services/autoformation/ipsa.htm>* **2002**
- *Internationale Bibliographie der geistes- und sozialwissenschaftlichen Zeitschriftenliteratur. . . See IBZ* **2002**
- *Journal of Social Work Practice "Abstracts Section" <http://www.carfax.co.uk/jsw-ad.htm>* **2002**
- *Links@Ovid (via CrossRef targeted DOI links) <http://www.ovid.com>* **2005**
- *National Adoption Information Clearinghouse Documents Database <http://naic.acf.hhs.gov>* **2002**
- *OCLC Public Affairs Information Service <http://www.pais.org>* . . . **2002**
- *OT SEARCH <http://www.aota.orglotsearch/>* **2002**
- *Ovid Linksolver (Open URL link resolver via CrossRef targeted DOI links) <http://www.linksolver.com>* **2005**
- *Peace Research Abstracts Journal* **2004**
- *Scopus (Elsevier) <http://www.info.scopus.com>* **2005**
- *Social Services Abstracts <http://www.csa.com>* **2003**
- *Social Work Abstracts <http://www.silverplatter.com/catalog/swab.htm>* **2003**
- *Violence and Abuse Abstracts: A Review of Current Literature on Interpersonal Violence (VAA)* **2002**

(continued)

Special Bibliographic Notes related to special journal issues (separates) and indexing/abstracting:

- indexing/abstracting services in this list will also cover material in any "separate" that is co-published simultaneously with Haworth's special thematic journal issue or DocuSerial. Indexing/abstracting usually covers material at the article/chapter level.
- monographic co-editions are intended for either non-subscribers or libraries which intend to purchase a second copy for their circulating collections.
- monographic co-editions are reported to all jobbers/wholesalers/approval plans. The source journal is listed as the "series" to assist the prevention of duplicate purchasing in the same manner utilized for books-in-series.
- to facilitate user/access services all indexing/abstracting services are encouraged to utilize the co-indexing entry note indicated at the bottom of the first page of each article/chapter/contribution.
- this is intended to assist a library user of any reference tool (whether print, electronic, online, or CD-ROM) to locate the monographic version if the library has purchased this version but not a subscription to the source journal.
- individual articles/chapters in any Haworth publication are also available through the Haworth Document Delivery Service (HDDS).

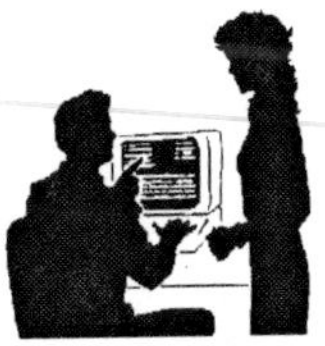

Cutting-Edge Social Policy Research

CONTENTS

ABOUT THE EDITOR

Richard Hoefer, PhD, is Associate Professor, School of Social Work, University of Texas at Arlington, Arlington, TX. He specializes in the areas of social policy and program administration, with a particular emphasis on advocacy and program evaluation. Dr. Hoefer is the founding editor of *The Social Policy Journal.* He is the author of *Advocacy Practice for Social Justice* and numerous articles on topics such as advocacy, nonprofit management, and program evaluation.

∞ ALL HAWORTH BOOKS AND JOURNALS
ARE PRINTED ON CERTIFIED
ACID-FREE PAPER

Preface

The manuscripts selected for this double issue of *The Social Policy Journal* emerged from the papers and presentations at the Social Policy Conference hosted by the University of South Carolina in 2004. As is often true of conference papers, the translation to a publishable article can be long and require considerable adaptation of the initial paper. In this case, the reviewers have done an excellent job of assisting, by their comments, and the authors have put additional efforts into what they may have thought were completed manuscripts. The product is one that all can be proud of.

Most impressive to me are the variety in approaches to the study of policy, the breadth of topics pursued and the number of younger scholars who are learning to write at the high level of expectations demanded by their academic colleagues sitting on the editorial review board. It bodes well for the profession of social work that all of these are true.

Terry Carrilio opens the collection with a discussion of what is in the "black box" of program implementation. The article provides an important contribution to measuring the extent to which a program has been implemented as planned, a step vital to making recommendations to policy makers. Linking program evaluation and policy practice in this way assists in remembering how practice and policy are interconnected.

Katherine H. Leith and Lyn Phillips, in the second article, provide the views of clients "in their own voices" to policy-makers. They argue that the results of qualitative approaches to policy research should be included in policy debates because such results are easier to read and more convincing to decision-makers.

[Haworth co-indexing entry note]: "Preface." Hoefer, Richard. Co-published simultaneously in *The Social Policy Journal* (The Haworth Press, Inc.) Vol. 4, No. 3/4, 2005, pp. xvii-xix; and:*Cutting-Edge Social Policy Research* (ed: Richard Hoefer) The Haworth Press, Inc., 2005, pp. xiii-xv Single or multiple copies of this article are available for a fee from The Haworth Document Delivery Service [1-800-HAWORTH, 9:00 a.m. - 5:00 p.m. (EST). E-mail address: docdelivery@haworthpress.com].

Available online at http://www.haworthpress.com/web/SPJ

doi:10.1300/J185v04n03_01

Another manuscript that uses clients' own words to inform decision-makers has been written by Kathryn McKinley and Geri Adler. Focusing on elderly persons in nursing homes, these authors provide a fascinating account of what matters to the quality of life of clients inside these institutions.

The next paper, by Emilie Edwards, Jennie Vaughn, and Karen Smith Rotabi, examines a population that cannot "speak for itself" in the typical way: deaf children. Demonstrating the higher levels of vulnerability that this population faces, the authors make a strong case for increased attention to ethical treatment and policy for these children.

Barbra A. Teater and David C. Kondrat next explicitly connect policy to practice in their examination of the Section 8 Housing program. The authors identify eight key variables of the Section 8 housing program, which leads to "an understanding of the program as a whole, the impact of the policy process on the recipients of the program, and the impact on social work practice." Generalizing these variables from housing to other policy arenas can provide social workers in all fields of practice a useful approach to understanding policy in their area.

Shawn A. Cassiman provides another conceptual paper. The argument made here is that a "trauma perspective" is helpful in understanding the true effects of poverty, inequality, and oppression in our society. Such a framework provides a needed alternative to a culture of poverty approach which is inherently individualistic in nature.

The next paper from the conference moves from qualitative and conceptual approaches to studying policy. Kyoung Hag Lee presents information on the effects of work incentive policies on clients in a rural and largely low-income state, West Virgina. This exacting quantitative manuscript shows clearly the power of numbers in illuminating the effects of social policy on clients.

The last manuscript in this volume is by Christopher Blanchard and Daniel D. Huff. Titled "Shadow Welfare II: Tax Expenditures and Corporate Welfare in the States," it is a companion article to one published in 2003 regarding federal tax policy. Information, such as in this paper, underscores the need for social workers to understand tax policy and economics as they make efforts to protect the remaining elements of the social welfare system.

The (almost) annual Policy Conference at which these papers were first presented represents a unique place for researchers to present their latest findings. Not only is there a ready-made audience of kindred spirits but the "after-presentation" and late night discussions that occur only when people are face-to-face are the genesis of additional thoughts and research ideas. It is my hope to attend many more Policy Conferences and to be able to reap the benefits of these gatherings of some of the best policy scholars in the country. Not only do the cutting-edge papers represent a treasure trove of information, but the friendships and camaraderie inspire me to continue thinking, researching, and writing about social policy.

Richard Hoefer, PhD
Editor

Looking Inside the "Black Box": A Methodology for Measuring Program Implementation and Informing Social Services Policy Decisions

Terry Carrilio

SUMMARY. The continued devolution of social welfare systems and services in the U.S. results in high stakes program evaluations in the field of family support and early intervention. Programs are expected to utilize evidence-based interventions and to demonstrate effectiveness. A look at implementation helps to differentiate between theories that do not work and programs that are not effective. Methods for identifying program implementation are needed. In a 17-site program evaluation, the author and her colleagues developed a methodology for measuring

---

Terry Carrilio, PhD, is affiliated with the San Diego State University, School of Social Work.

Address correspondence to: Terry Carrilio, PhD, San Diego State University, School of Social Work, 5500 Campanile Drive, San Diego, CA 92182-4119 (E-mail: tbear10009@aol.com).

A version of this paper was presented at The Policy Conference: "Social Policy Change in a Polarized Nation," August 7-10, 2004, Charleston, SC.

[Haworth co-indexing entry note]: "Looking Inside the 'Black Box': A Methodology for Measuring Program Implementation and Informing Social Services Policy Decisions." Carrilio, Terry. Co-published simultaneously in *The Social Policy Journal* (The Haworth Press, Inc.) Vol. 4, No. 3/4, 2005, pp. 1-17; and: *Cutting-Edge Social Policy Research* (ed: Richard Hoefer) The Haworth Press, Inc., 2005, pp. 1-17. Single or multiple copies of this article are available for a fee from The Haworth Document Delivery Service [1-800-HAWORTH, 9:00 a.m. - 5:00 p.m. (EST). E-mail address: docdelivery@haworthpress.com].

Available online at http://www.haworthpress.com/web/SPJ

doi:10.1300/J185v04n03_01

implementation and demonstrated the effects of differential implementation in understanding program outcomes.

KEYWORDS. Program evaluation, program implementation, evidence-based practice, model fidelity, outcomes

This paper will discuss the importance of identifying program implementation factors that affect the evaluation of program effectiveness, particularly at a time when social policy discussions are questioning whether many programs are necessary at all (O'Connor, 2001; Twombly, 2002). After a brief overview of how this discussion has emerged in the field of family support, a method for examining program implementation will be presented with an example of its application in a seventeen-site evaluation.

MEASURING PROGRAM IMPLEMENTATION IS URGENT IN A POLARIZED POLICY ENVIRONMENT

The American social welfare system has been undergoing a process of "devolution" in which programs and attitudes towards those needing support and assistance are undergoing fundamental changes (Pandey & Collier-Tenison, 2001; Weiss, 2001). This devolution involves reducing the federal role in addressing the social well being of the population, and placing more and more fiscal burden upon states, local governments, and voluntary organizations (Whitaker & Time, 2001). The focus on religion and "family values" demonstrates a growing belief by many that the responsibility for managing social and personal vulnerabilities is a private one, and the public responsibility is more and more limited to areas of social control and defense. Current trends towards developing "faith-based" services represent a return to early residual models of social welfare (Marwell, 2004; Whitaker & Time, 2001). A paradoxical debate ensues in which well-meaning people are encouraged to provide the needed supports for the most vulnerable members of society, while distrust of professional helpers increases. The underlying social contract, operational since the mid 1930s, between individuals and the community, as represented by formal programs of support, has been undergoing a long process of deconstruction (O'Connor, 2001; Weiss, 2001). Current trends towards the use of informal, rather than formal support systems reflect a belief that public responsibility for well being should be reduced, and that reliance on the family should be increased (Eisenberg & Carrilio, 1983; Pandey & Collier-Tenison, 2001). If the family unit is overburdened or not functioning well, in a context in which formal social supports have been reduced and more demands are placed upon the family, individuals, particularly children, may be at risk of preventable adverse circumstances.

While a sense of public support for vulnerable families has decreased, burdens on families have increased. The field of family support has sought to identify effective methods for strengthening families. In an environment in which professional programs are considered equal to or even less valid than religious and voluntary programs (Hodge, 2003; Twombly, 2002), the demand for demonstrating effects plays a powerful role in program development and evaluation (Carrilio, 2003; Proctor, 2002; Witkin & Harrison, 2001). The movement in the helping professions towards evidence-based practice reflects a trend in the development of professional practice as well as a new resource in determining where and how to utilize social welfare resources (Cournoyer, 2004; Gambrill, 2003; Webb, 2002). This paper explores the importance of including an examination of program implementation in understanding program effectiveness, and suggests that a focus on program implementation be included in the development of policies and services addressing the needs of vulnerable families.

FAMILY SUPPORT PROGRAMS IN A POLARIZED ENVIRONMENT

The field of family support occupies an interesting junction of sometimes conflicting paradigms regarding the degree and amount of intervention that is necessary to maintain a healthy society. Bolstering both common sense and the traditional "person-in-environment" perspective of social work, recent research into resilience and vulnerability indicates that the context of early childhood profoundly influences later outcomes (Buka & Earls, 1993; Erickson & Kurtz-Reimer, 1999; Illig, 1998; Kotulak, 1995; Reynolds et al., 2001).

The focus on the early context of development is the family, and the context within which the family is carrying out its functions (Garbarino,

1995; Schorr & Schorr, 1988; Shonkoff & Phillips, 2000). Practitioners, policy makers, and researchers have observed that poverty, community violence, and other aspects of the community context adversely affect families (Garbarino, 1995; Knitzer, 1999; Shokoff & Phillips, 2000). The paradigm that emerges from these observations is one that recognizes the need for a society to invest in its children by investing in families and communities (Guterman, 2001; Karoly, 1998). This type of thinking leads advocates to encourage supportive services for all families, not only those who have been identified as 'at risk' (Krugman, 1993). The investment paradigm tends to be preventive and focuses on building capacities in individuals, families, organizations, and communities.

A powerful competing paradigm that has gained credibility over the past quarter century is the moral/religious paradigm. Following this framework, it is expected that individuals and families take responsibility for their own problems and expect help from the larger society only as a last resort. This approach puts problems into a moral or religious framework, and suggests to the sufferer that individual salvation will result in an improved situation (Hodge, 2003, O'Connor, 2001; Weiss, 2001). This paradigm suggests intervention from entities outside of the family only after family resources have broken down. Recently it has led to an intrusion into defining families and the "values" that are expected by the larger social system. It is not the topic of this paper, but one of the disturbing offshoots of this thinking is the preference for using public resources to monitor morality rather than for mitigating the powerful social and economic forces affecting families.

In the face of these different views on what families need, family support programs are pressed to demonstrate efficacy. Policy makers seek "silver bullets." They want research evidence that demonstrates conclusively that the programs they fund "work" (Horsch, 1996; Julian & Clapp, 2000; Poertner, 2000; Schorr, 1997). However, defining what "works" is complicated. Family support is a complex concept that incorporates intervention at the client level, the organizational level, and the community level (Carrilio, 2001; Carrilio et al., 2002; Garbarino, 1995; Gomby et al., 1999). Recent efforts to find results from these programs have been mixed (Carrilio, 2003; Chafin, 2004; Duggan et al., 1999; Gomby, 1999; Landsverk et al., 2002; Olds et al., 2002; Stratham & Holtermann, 2004). It is possible that the logic models of many family support programs do not adequately address specific risk factors (Bugental et al., 2002; Chafin, 2004). From a policy standpoint this is disturbing because without clear "silver bullets," the discussion of how to effectively enhance family functioning can easily deteriorate into a paradigm war, with each side claiming evidence for its perspective. For this reason, it is incumbent upon program developers, policy makers, practitioners and researchers to carefully understand the underlying purposes of programs and what actually takes place in programs in order to understand what is and is not working (Daro & Harding, 1999; Harachi, 1999; Simmel, 2002; Stratham & Holtermann, 2004; Tidmarsh & Carpenter, 2003). In the current polarized policy context this is not an academic discussion; it has consequences for how programs are funded and what those programs are expected to accomplish.

Model family support programs which have shown promise often produce disappointing results when they are taken "to scale" (Gomby, 1999; Gomby et al., 1999; Schorr, 1997). One interpretation of the somewhat disappointing showing of many prevention efforts might be that there has been an implementation failure, which in turn affects the outcomes of the program. (Duggan et al., 1999; Duggan et al., 2004; Gomby et al., 1999; Harachi et al., 1999; Rossi, Freeman & Lipsey, 1999; Straw & Herrell, 2002). Another possibility is that the underlying conceptual base of the program is inadequate or poorly articulated (Chafin, 2004; Clapp & Early, 1999; Rossi et al., 1999). Practitioners, researchers, and policy makers need to address the need for consistent results through systematic program design, research, and implementation.

CAPTURING IMPLEMENTATION DATA

Implementation is a key component in understanding program outcomes (Carrilio, 2003; Jerrell & Ridgely, 1999; Orwin, 2000; Rossi et al., 1999; Straw & Herrell, 2002). Ideology and agency context strongly affect the ways that program innovations will be integrated into practice (Burke & Clapp, 1997; Carrilio et al., 2003; Hodges & Hernandez, 1999). Program design, implementation and evaluation are closely related (Hogue, 1996; Julian & Clapp, 2000; Teague, 1998; Tidmarsh et al., 2003). Evaluation methods that use a "black box" approach often present a two dimensional picture of program effectiveness (Copeland & Wexler, 1995; Donaldson & Scriven, 2003; Harachi et al., 1999) and fail to adequately account for the organizational and community context within which the intervention is taking place.

While there is growing recognition of the need to take program implementation into account in understanding program outcomes, methodologies for examining implementation need to be developed (Domitrovich & Greenberg, 2000; Everhart & Wandersman, 2000; Jerrell & Ridgely, 1999; Leff & Mulkern, 2002; Teague, 1998; Vinson, 2001). A number of authors point out that beyond measures of implementation it is important to also look at "treatment adherence" (Hogue, 1996; Orwin, 2000; Teague, 1998; Vinson, 2001). This refers to the degree to which the intervention as suggested by theory is actually carried out. Treatment adherence begins to approach the question of "quality" (Domitrovich & Greenberg, 2000; Jerrell & Ridgely, 1999; Rossi et al., 1999), which is key to understanding program-level effectiveness and participant-level outcomes.

Despite the common sense and research support for connecting underlying program theory and values with program activities (Hernandez, 2000), in the real world of social policy and program funding it is often the case that program staff are not clear on how the program elements relate to an underlying theory (Clapp & Early, 1999; Julian & Clapp, 2000). As a result, day-to-day decisions in the program are often made on the basis of expediency and individual ideologies. Often programs are designed at the policy level, funded, operationalized, and evaluated without sufficient recognition that the program-as-implemented may have deviated significantly from the original premises of the program-as-designed (Duggan et al., 1999; Gomby, 1999; Harachi, 1999; Jerrell & Ridgely, 1999; Straw & Herrel, 2002). Additionally, in a volatile policy environment, it is possible for the funding agencies to actually change their underlying assumptions mid-project (Carrilio et al., 2002; Carrilio, 2003). Yet, program evaluations often proceed somewhat mechanically, assuming that the intervention has gone as planned, and has provided the requisite services in the dosage, manner, and intensity called for in the original logic model, if one has been made explicit (Domitrivich & Greenberg, 2000; Orwin, 2000; Teague, 1998).

This "black box" approach assumes that there are resources, system support, organizational and staff capacity, and leadership focused on an agreed upon logic model and set of expectations about how the program should operate. There can be considerable variance among and within program sites with respect to how they believe their work connects to the underlying program logic model (Harachi et al., 1999; Jerrell & Ridgely, 1999; Orwin, 1999; Simmel, 2002; Tidmarsh et al., 2003; Vinson, 2001). In prior research the author and colleagues have found that attitudinal factors play a role in how program expectations are understood and acted upon by staff and administrators (Carrilio et al., 2003).

In multi-site projects, which are common when funders are seeking to develop programs that reflect policy imperatives, differential implementation both within and between sites must be accounted for in any discussion of the program's effectiveness (Straw & Herrell, 2002; Vinson, 2001).

In a recent multi-site evaluation the authors and colleagues developed a model of program design, implementation and evaluation (Carrilio, in press) as described in Figure 1.

As illustrated in the model, implementation includes both client-level and organizational components, as well as recognition of the community and policy context within which a program is taking place. The following methodological outline serves as a way to measure and utilize program implementation as a tool in the evaluation and policy-making process:

1. *Logic Model:* A program logic model should be articulated and clarified with stakeholders, including the program funder and the service providers prior to the initiation of services.

FIGURE 1. Model of Program Design, Implementation, and Evaluation

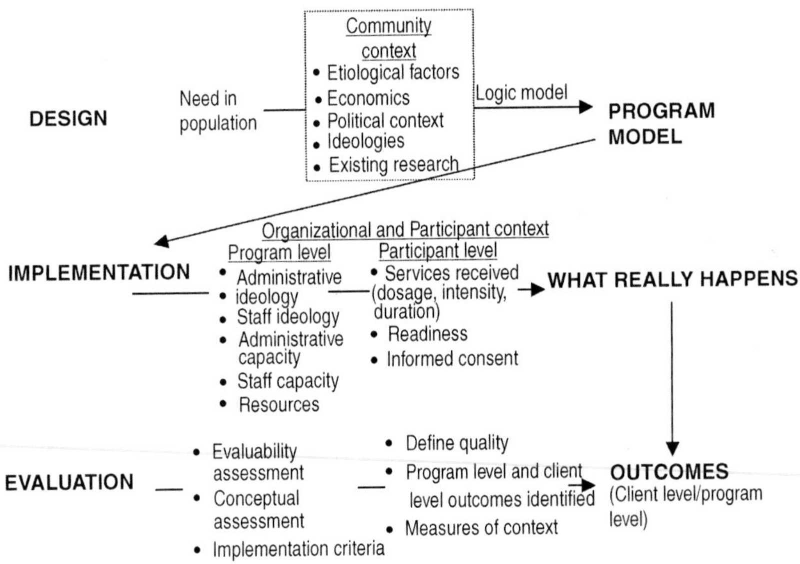

2. *Program Implementation Checklist:* Using the logic model, a checklist breaking down every specific program component needed in order to provide program activities that support the theoretical model needs to be developed. Additionally, stakeholders at the policy/funding, organizational, community, and client level should be aware of the checklist.
3. *Identification of Implementation Domains and Measures:* Using the logic model and program implementation checklist the stakeholders and the research team should identify the measures that will demonstrate that, in fact, the specified activities are taking place. Frequently this will involve identifying key domains of implementation, such as "agency context," "services delivered," and so on. The domains should include data at the client, staff, organizational, community, and policy level.
4. *Data Collection:* A strategy for collecting the data for each domain needs to be established, ideally, prior to initiating the program.
5. *Evaluation of Program Outcomes Taking Implementation into Account:* Using the logic model, expected outcomes at the client, organizational, community, and policy level should be assessed, taking into account the level of program implementation that can be demonstrated by using the domains developed at step 3.
6. *Program and Policy Integration:* The results at the client, organizational, community, and policy level should be analyzed with the original logic model in mind. Questions about whether the logic model was robust enough, along with recommendations for making adjustments based on the new evidence are key to this step. The understanding of what the results mean and how they can be used in future program development would ideally be used to initiate a new round of program development and refinement.

Figure 2 illustrates this methodology and its role in the policy-making process.

CASE EXAMPLE–MEASURING IMPLEMENTATION AND ITS IMPACT ON A 17-SITE PROGRAM EVALUATION

From July 1999 though June 2001, the California Department of Social Services funded a comprehensive family support demonstration project in seventeen California counties. The project was the outgrowth

FIGURE 2. Measuring Implementation in a Policy and Program Development Context

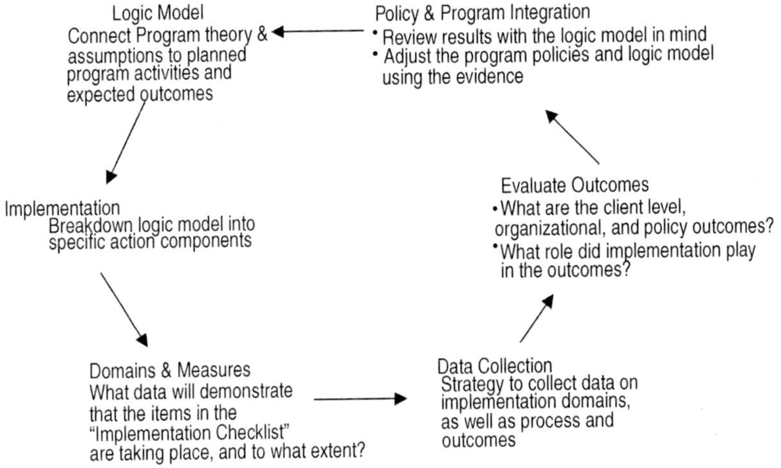

of two previous program policy initiatives (Carrilio, 2003) and relied heavily on the evaluation findings and recommendations from the two prior projects as well as new findings appearing in the professional literature (Gomby et al., 1999; Karoly et al., 1998; Schorr, 1997; Yoshikowa, 1995). The policy goal of this complex program was to integrate the emerging evidence on home visiting and family resource centers as effective means of providing community-based primary prevention and early intervention for vulnerable families. Additionally, the funder, a state agency, was interested in promoting an ideology of prevention in child welfare and planned to develop integrated center-based and home-based programs at the county level.

The vicissitudes of implementing this project (Carrilio et al., under review; Carrilio et al., 2003) led the evaluators to observe that understanding this project required examining the interactions among three layers of information: (1) the policy/funder layer; (2) the outcomes proposed in the logic model; (3) the effects of implementation. At the policy/funder level changes in leadership and conflicting policy agendas at the funding agency resulted in inconsistent guidance to the project sites. Many of the projects came in with their own ideological perspectives and were less interested in implementing the program's theoretical model than in receiving funds for existing operations. An additional factor at the policy/funder level was the trendy, but poorly articulated, demand that each site involve multi-organizational collaboration in carrying out the project. Important factors such as differences in organizational cultures, salaries, and benefits were powerful barriers for sites (Carrilio et al., 2002).

At the outcomes level, the staffs at the funding organization and at the sites implementing the program were confused about the level at which to focus their energies. The logic model called for outcomes at the client, community and policy levels. However, because of conflicting agendas entering into the project and unclear leadership from the funder, the logic model was poorly understood and did not play a significant role for the funders or the program sites. As reported elsewhere (Carrilio et al., 2003), this resulted in insufficient data to assess client-level outcomes. Process data were available, and we were able to assess some of the community-level outcome. Additionally, as a result of leadership changes at the policy/funding agency, by the end of the project the original concern for client-level outcomes was almost non-existent and the staff reading the report were primarily interested in larger policy questions that had not been part of the initial design.

Shifting policy messages and the resulting confusion in the logic model strongly influenced the implementation of the project. Early in the evaluation process the research team recognized the need to measure implementation. The first two steps in the suggested methodology for measuring implementation had been followed. Stakeholders were aware of both the logic model and the program implementation checklist. Despite this, the research staff identified noticeable differences in how the program was being implemented across sites (Carrilio et al., 2002; Carrilio, in press). In order to capture these differences, the research team initiated the third step, which involved the identification of eight implementation domains and measures that would reflect those domains. Specific program and data elements were identified for each domain. The program implementation checklist was used as a standard of comparison and the degree to which each site met or deviated from the standard was rated. For each domain there were multiple elements rated, and finally, all of the elements for the domain were combined to create an overall score for that domain. Sites received a score for each of the 8 domains and a summary score for overall implementation.

The strategy for collecting data involved gathering both quantitative and qualitative data at the client, staff, program administration, organizational, and community levels. Client and staff level service delivery data were collected on a daily basis through a computerized management information system. There were three cycles of on-site data collection involving the administration of survey instruments, interviews, and program observations at the client, staff, program administration, and community levels. These data were used to extract the domain scores.

The analysis of the data from the management information system and the site visits was used to understand the program's effectiveness and impact. The results were mixed. At the program level, we found that some aspects of the program design, such as the introduction of integrated teams, the requirement that staff receive regular training, and that services be integrated into family resource centers, achieved between 84-88 percent of full implementation. Through interviews and observations, it was evident that the program had encouraged more collaboration, the use of multi-level, integrated teams, and an integration of center-based and home based services. The results on the program's impact in the local communities were promising as well, with an overall domain score of 79 percent implementation. Interviews and surveys indicated that there had been some realignment of thinking in the local communities towards prevention and better integration of resources.

However, we also found that organizational culture and client outcomes were less encouraging. At the organizational level we found barriers associated with lack of administrative skill and poor management of human resources. The data indicate that efforts at collaboration both within and across agencies were negatively affected by differences in salaries among staff doing similar work. Actual services to clients were poorly implemented, with the services domain only demonstrating 40 percent of full implementation. At the client level, while we were able to capture process data through the management information system, client-level outcomes were hard to identify because programs complied poorly with the administration of the standardized measures that were supposed to track client progress. Additionally, services were not provided at the intensity or for the duration specified by the logic model.

In summary, the results indicated the following:

1. The program as specified in the logic model and the program implementation checklist were only partially implemented. Two key areas of concern were in the area of service delivery to clients and the human resources/organizational context.
2. Implementation was affected by the leadership and community contexts within which programs were operating.
3. Implementation was negatively impacted by lack of clarity and changing priorities at the funding/policy level.

4. The failure to implement parts of the program-as-designed affected our ability to assess client-level outcomes and left many of the questions about what constituted "best practices" unanswered.

In keeping with the final step in the outline for utilizing implementation in program evaluation described above, a report was presented to the funders and shared with each site. The researchers initiated a dialogue with the funders and the program sites to review the project and identify recommendations for more successful implementation in the future. Because of changed policy priorities and because most of the program sites were scrambling to find continued funding, the integrative process suggested in the final step was abbreviated. While it would be ideal to have all stakeholders review the original program design, examine how it was implemented and what the results were, and develop program enhancements and refinements on the basis of this information, in a high stakes policy environment this is unlikely. However, it is important that programs working with vulnerable families operate with the best information so that they can enhance positive outcomes and reduce adverse outcomes. For this reason, one of the "lessons learned" from this project has been the importance of defining the entire process at the beginning and achieving commitment from stakeholders to complete the process.

CONCLUSIONS

The example above illustrates the way in which implementation played a role in understanding the effectiveness of a policy-driven program in a volatile policy environment. The actual program model and imperatives changed over the course of the project. The demands of good evaluation and evidence-based practice require a systematic, clearly articulated process that undergoes review and careful refinement and adjustment with new information. On the other hand, the world of policy makers and funders is more driven by trends, the search for quick fixes and silver bullets, and the need to change course with political winds. In this context, simply carrying out an evaluation that studies client and program outcomes in a static manner can be misleading, and even destructive, if implementation is not taken into account.

As programs are scrutinized more closely and pressure increases to produce "results," the policy debates tend to focus on which program "models" are the most effective (Chafin, 2004; Gomby et al., 1999; Schorr, 1997; Teague, 1998; Tidmarsh et al., 2003; Webb, 2002). However, it is possible that rather than trying to find the right "off the shelf" model, policy makers and program staff should be educated to attend closely to the specifics of implementation and program operations. It is important to distinguish between a model that does not meet the need and a specific implementation that may not be true to the theoretical model (Rossi et al., 1999). The 17 sites described above all believed that they were following "the model," yet our data show vast differences in how the programs were actually operating. Data from interviews at the staff, administrative, and community levels indicate considerable variance in attitudes toward, and understanding of, the model among different players at each site, and between sites (Carrilio et al., 2002). It is noteworthy that this variance was observed despite intensive pre-implementation staff training and regular feedback sessions with program staff and administrators (Carrilio et al., 2003).

In the example above, without looking at the differential implementation not only across sites, but across program content domains, it would have been easy to conclude that family support programs for vulnerable families are not effective (Chafin, 2004; Duggan, 2004; Gomby, 1999; Guterman, 2001; Landsverk et al., 2002; Olds, 1999; Stratham & Holtermann, 2004). However, by looking at how the program was implemented at each site, it is clear that in order to identify program effects, one has to carry out the program-as-designed. In the case example, a key component of the program, the services to clients, were inconsistently implemented. Our study of implementation provided some insight into how the program became diluted and in what ways. In designing multi-site projects, planners would be well-advised to carefully attend to both the robustness of the proposed model and to the fine balance between maintaining centralized control over implementation and encouraging local input and adaptations. Future work building upon the outline for a method to identify key factors influencing implementation described in this paper can play an important part in developing evidence-based policies and programs for vulnerable families.

REFERENCES

Bugental, D. B., Ellerson, P. C., Lin, E. K., Rainey, B., Kokotovic, A., & O'Hara, N. (2002). A cognitive approach to child abuse prevention. *Journal of Family Psychology, 16*(3), 243-258.

Buka, S., & Earls, F. (1993). Early determinants of delinquency and violence. *Health Affairs, 12*(4), 46-64.

Burke, A. C., & Clapp, J. D. (1997). Ideology and social work practice in substance abuse settings. *Social Work, 42*(6), 552-562.

Carrilio, T. (1998). *California Safe and Healthy Families: Executive Summary* (2nd Ed.). Sacramento: California Department of Social Services.

Carrilio, T. (2001). Family support program development-integrating research, practice, and policy. *Journal of Family Social Work, 6*(3), 53-78.

Carrilio, T., Packard, T., Cannady, L., Darling, M., Chamberlin, J., Gamble, L., Bergthold, T., & Dorosky, E. (2002). *Final report–Answers Benefitting Children program evaluation.* Technical report submitted to the California Department of Social Services Office of Child Abuse Prevention.

Carrilio, T., Packard, T., & Clapp, J. (2003). Nothing in-nothing out: Barriers to the use of performance data in social service programs. *Administration in Social Work, 27*(4), 61-75.

Carrilio, T. (2003). Learning from experience? A review of three California initiatives addressing the needs of vulnerable families. *Social Policy Journal, 2*(2/3), 5-25.

Carrilio, T. (in press). The elusive search for the silver bullet in prevention and family support programs for vulnerable families. *Social Work and Social Sciences Review.*

Chafin, M. (2004). Is it time to re-think Healthy Start/Healthy Families? *Child Abuse & Neglect, 28*(6), 589-595.

Clapp, J. D., & Early, T. J. (1999). A qualitative exploratory study of substance abuse prevention outcomes in a heterogeneous prevention system. *Journal of Drug Education, 29*(3), 217-233.

Cournoyer, B. (2004). *The evidence-based social work skills book.* New York: Allyn & Bacon.

Daro. D., & Harding, K. (1999). Healthy Families America: Using research to enhance practice. In Behrman, R. (Ed.), *The future of children: Recent program evaluations, 9*(1). David and Lucille Packard Foundation, 152-176.

Domitrovich, C. E., & Greenberg, M. T. (2000). The study of implementation: Current findings from effective programs that prevent mental disorders in school-aged children. *Journal of Educational & Psychological Consultation, 11*(2), 93-221.

Donaldson, S. I., & Scriven, M. (2003). *Evaluating social programs and problems.* Mahwah, NJ: Lawrence Erlbaum Associates.

Duggan, A., McFarlane, E., Fuddy, L., Burrell, L., Higman, S. M., Winham, A., & Sia, C. (2004). Randomized trial of a statewide home visiting program: Impact in preventing child abuse and neglect. *Child Abuse & Neglect, 28*(6), 597-622.

Duggan, A., McFarlane, E., Windham, A., Rohde, C., Salkever, D., Fuddy, L., Rosenberg, L., Buchbinder, S., & Sia, C. (1999). Evaluation of Hawaii's Healthy Start Program in Behrman, R. (Ed.), *The future of children: Recent program evaluations, 9*(1). David and Lucille Packard Foundation, 66-90.

Eisenberg, D., & Carrilio, T. (1983). Informal resources for the elderly: Panacea or empty promise? *Journal of Gerontological Social Work, 6*(1), 39-47.

Erikson, M., & Kurz-Reimer, K. (1999). *Infants, toddlers, and families: A framework for support and intervention.* New York: The Guilford Press.

Everhart, K., & Wandersman, A. (2000). Applying comprehensive quality programming and empowerment evaluation to reduce implementation barriers. *Journal of Educational & Psychological Consultation, 11*(2), 177-191.

Gambrill, E.D. (2003). Evidence-based practice: Sea change or the emperor's new clothes? *Journal of Social Work Education, 39*(1), 3-23.

Garbarino, J. (1995). *Raising children in a socially toxic environment.* San Francisco: Jossey-Bass.

Gomby, D., Culross, P., & Behrman, R. (1999). Home visiting: Recent program evaluations–Analysis and recommendations. In Behrman, R. (Ed.), *The future of children: Recent program evaluations, 9*(1). David and Lucille Packard Foundation, 4-26.

Gomby, D. (1999). Understanding evaluations of home visitation programs. In Behrman, R. (Ed.), *The future of children: Recent program evaluations, 9*(1). David and Lucille Packard Foundation, 27-43.

Guterman, N. B. (2001). *Stopping child maltreatment before it starts.* Thousand Oaks, CA: Sage Publications.

Harachi, T. W., Abbott, R. D., Catalano, R. F., Haggerty, K. P., & Fleming, C. B. (1999). Opening the black box: Using process evaluation measures to assess implementation and theory building. *American Journal of Community Psychology, 27*(5), 711-731.

Hernandez, M. (2000). Using logic models and program theory to build outcome accountability. *Education and Treatment of Children, 23*(1), 24-40.

Hodge, D. R. (2003). Differences in worldviews between social workers and people of faith. *Families in Society, 84*(2), 285-295.

Hodges, S., & Hernandez, M. (1999). How organizational culture influences outcome information utilization. *Evaluation and Program Planning, 22*(2), 183-197.

Hogue, A. (1996). Treatment adherence process research in family therapy: A rationale and some practical guidelines. *Psychotherapy, 33*(2), 332-345.

Horsch, K. (1996). Results-based accountability systems: Opportunities and challenges. *The Evaluation Exchange, 2*(1), 2-3. Electronic journal published by The Harvard Family Research Project, retrieved on April 30, 2005 from *http://www.gse.harvard.edu/hfrp/eval.html.*

Illig, D. (1998). *Birth to kindergarten: The importance of the early years.* California State Library Monograph No. CR-98-001. Sacramento: California Research Bureau.

Jerrell, J., & Ridgely, M. (1999). The relative impact of treatment program robustness and dosage. *Evaluation and Program Planning, 22*(3), 323-330.

Julian, D., & Clapp, J. D. (2000). Outcomes based funding and the logic model: Mechanisms for coordinating human services at the local level. *Evaluation and Program Planning, 23*(2), 231-240.

Kagen, S. L., & Neville, P. (1993). *Integrating services for children and families.* New Haven: Yale University Press.

Karoly, L. Greenwood, P., Evringham, S., Hoube, J., Kilburn, M. R., Rydell, P., Saunders, M., & Chiesa, J. (1998). *Investing in our children: What we know and don't know about the costs and benefits of early childhood interventions.* Rand MR 898-TCWF. Santa Monica: Rand Corporation.

Knitzer, J. (1999). *Promoting resiliency among the most stressed young children and families: Toward more responsive welfare-linked policies and programs.* The National Center for Children in Poverty. Joseph L. Mailman School of Public Health. Columbia University.

Kotulak, R. (1995). *Inside the brain: Revolutionary discoveries of how the mind works.* Kansas City: Andrews and McMeel.

Krugman, R. (1993). Universal home visiting: A recommendation from the U.S. Advisory Board on Child Abuse and Neglect. In Behrman, R. (Ed.), *The future of children: Home visiting, 3*(3). David and Lucille Packard Foundation, 184-191.

Landsverk, J., Carrilio, T. E., Connelly, C. D., Ganger, W. C., Slymen, D. J., Newton, R. R., & Jones, C. (2002). *Healthy Families San Diego clinical trial: Technical report.* San Diego Children's Hospital and Health Center, Child and Adolescent Services Research Center.

Leff, H. S., & Mulkern, V. (2002). Lessons learned about science and participation from multisite evaluations. In J.M. Herrell & R.B. Straw (Eds.), *New Directions for Evaluation, 94.* San Francisco: Jossey-Bass, 89-100.

Marwell, N. P. (2004). Privatizing the welfare state: Nonprofit community-based organizations as political actors. *American Sociological Review, 69*(2), 265-291.

O'Connor, B. (2001). The protagonists and ideas behind the Personal Responsibility and Work Opportunity Reconciliation Act of 1996: The enactment of a conservative welfare system. *Social Justice, 28*(4), 4-32.

Olds, D., Henderson, C., Kitzman, H., Eckenrode, J., Cole, R., & Tattlebaum, R. (1999). Prenatal and infancy home visitation by nurses: Recent findings. In Behrman, R. (Ed.), *The future of children: Recent program evaluations, 9*(1). David and Lucille Packard Foundation, 44-63.

Olds, D. L., Robinson, J., O'Brien, R., Luckey, D. W., Pettit, L., Henderson, L., Jr., Ng, R., Sheff, K., Korfmacher, J., Hiat, S., & Talmi, A. (2002). Home visiting by paraprofessionals and by nurses: A randomized, controlled trial. *Pediatrics, 110*(3): 486-497.

Orwin, R. (2000). Assessing program fidelity in substance abuse health services research. *Addiction, 95*(supplement 13), S 309-S327.

Pandey, S., & Collier-Tenison, S. (2001). Welfare reform: An exploration of devolution. *Social Justice, 28*(1), 54-75.

Poertner, J. (2000). Managing for service outcomes. In R. Patti (Ed.), *The handbook of social welfare management.* Thousand Oaks, CA: Sage Publications, 267-281.

Proctor, E. K. (2002). Quality of care and social work research. *Social Work Research, 26*(4), 195-197.

Reynolds, A. J., Temple, J., Robertson, D., & Mann, E. (2001). Long term effects of an early childhood intervention on educational achievement and juvenile arrest: A 15-year follow-up of low-income children in public schools. *Journal of the American Medical Association, 285*(18), 2339-2346.

Rossi, P. H., Freman, H. E., & Lipsey, M. W. (1999). *Evaluation: A systematic approach* (6th ed.). Thousand Oaks, CA: Sage Publications.

Schorr, L., & Schorr, D. (1988). *Within our reach: Breaking the cycle of disadvantage.* New York: Anchor Books (Doubleday).

Schorr, L. (1997). *Common purpose: Strengthening families and neighborhoods to rebuild America.* New York: Doubleday.

Shonkoff, J. P., & Phillips, D. A. (2000). *From neurons to neighborhoods: The science of early childhood development.* National Research Council and Institute of Medicine Board on Children, Youth, and Families, Commission on Behavioral and Social Sciences and Education. Washington, DC: National Academy Press.

Simmel, C. (2002). The Shared Family Care development project: Challenges of implementing and evaluating a community based project. *Children and Youth Services Review, 24*(6-7), 455-470.

Stratham, J., & Holtermann, S. (2004). Families on the brink: The effectiveness of family support services. *Child & Family Social Work, 9*(2), 153-166.

Straw, R. B., & Herrell, J. M. (2002). A framework for understanding and improving multisite evaluations. In J.M. Herrell & R.B. Straw (Eds.), *New Directions for Evaluation, 94*. San Francisco: Jossey-Bass: 5-15.

Teague, G. (1998). Program fidelity in assertive community treatment: Development and use of a measure. *American Journal of Orthopsychiatry, 68*(2), 216-232.

Tidmarsh, J., Carpenter, J., & Slade, J. (2003). Practitioners as gatekeepers and researchers: Family support outcomes. *The International Journal of Sociology and Social Policy, 13*(1/2), 59-80.

Twombly, E. C. (2002). Religious versus secular human services organizations: Implications for public policy. *Social Science Quarterly, 83*(4), 947-961.

Vinson, N. (2001). The system of care model: Implementation in 27 communities. *Journal of Emotional & Behavioral Disorders, 9*(1), 30-42.

Webb, S. (2002). Evidence-based practice and decision analysis in social work: An implementation model. *Journal of Social Work, 2*(1), 45-63.

Weiss, R. P. (2001). Charitable choice as neoliberal social welfare strategy. *Social Justice, 28*(1), 35-54.

Whitaker, I. P., & Time, V. (2001). Devolution and welfare: The social and legal implications of state inequalities for welfare reform in the United States. *Social Justice, 28*(1), 76-90.

Witkin, S. L., & Harrison, W. D. (2001) Whose evidence and for what purpose? *Social Work, 46*(4), 293-296.

Yoshikawa, H. (1995). Long-term effects of early childhood programs on social outcomes and delinquency. In Behrman, R. (Ed.), *The future of children: Long term outcomes of early childhood programs. 5*(3). David and Lucille Packard Foundation, 51-70.

"In Their Own Voices": Using Qualitative Research and Consumer Narratives for Systems Change

Katherine H. Leith
Lyn Phillips

SUMMARY. Social policy should be informed by scientific research. Yet, the rapport between researchers and policy makers remains poor, and the translation of social research into social policy haphazard. Many researchers follow a positivist paradigm and prepare quantitative reports that are difficult for policy makers to decipher. Good research is "wasted" because policy makers consider it irrelevant to the real-life problems of their constituents. Policy research that are qualitative narratives are more reader-friendly and thus more appealing to policy makers. This article argues for the inclusion of qualitative

Katherine H. Leith, PhD, LMSW, and Lyn Phillips, LMSW, are affiliated with the Center for Health Services and Policy Research, Norman J. Arnold School of Public Health, University of South Carolina.

Address correspondence to: Katherine H. Leith, PhD, LMSW, Center for Health Services and Policy Research, University of South Carolina, Devine Street, Columbia, SC 29208 (E-mail: leith@sc.edu).

An earlier version of this article was presented at the 2004 annual Policy Conference on Politics, Policy, and Social Change in Charleston, SC.

[Haworth co-indexing entry note]: "'In Their Own Voices': Using Qualitative Research and Consumer Narratives for Systems Change." Leith, Katherine, H., and Lyn Phillips. Co-published simultaneously in *The Social Policy Journal* (The Haworth Press, Inc.) Vol. 4, No. 3/4, 2005, pp. 19-35; and: *Cutting-Edge Social Policy Research* (ed: Richard Hoefer) The Haworth Press, Inc., 2005, pp. 19-35. Single or multiple copies of this article are available for a fee from The Haworth Document Delivery Service [1-800-HAWORTH, 9:00 a.m. - 5:00 p.m. (EST). E-mail address: docdelivery@haworthpress.com].

Available online at http://www.haworthpress.com/web/SPJ

doi:10.1300/J185v04n03_02

methods into research conducted to inform social policy and offers several case examples.

KEYWORDS. Qualitative research, public policy, research-policy relationship

INTRODUCTION

Ideally, the policies and programs designed to address existing social problems should be driven by scientific research to ensure their viability (Black, 2001). Yet the literature suggests that the relationship between social sciences researchers and policy makers always has been, and remains, tenuous, and the dissemination of research into relevant policy slow and haphazard (Feldman, Nadash, & Gursen, 2001; Merrill & Somers, 1985; Rosenthal, 1981; Trostle, Bronfman, & Langer, 1999; Weiss, 1977). The "research to practice gap" is long-standing and well-documented (Carise, Cornely, & Gurel, 2002; Institute of Medicine, 1998). Moreover, it appears to be international (Davis & Howden- Chapman, 1996; Rozzini & Trabucchi, 2001; Trostle et al., 1999). For example, Trostle et al. (1999) discuss the findings of their recent study that point to a number of impediments to the use of research by health decision-makers in Mexico. Similarly, Rozzini and Trabucchi (2001) describe the communications between researchers and local government in Italy as "mercurial," with the responsibility for much of the friction generally being allocated to the researcher's side. In this country, Feldman et al. (2001) provide a detailed account of the complex nature of the relationship between researchers and policy makers in this the field of long-term care, from each side's respective point of view.

This article offers insight into the relationship between research and policy by framing it against the different paradigms that underlie each side. Drawing from the health research/health policy literature, it includes a discussion about various models of the nature of relationships between researchers and policy makers that reflect these paradigmatic differences and about concrete reasons for the poor translation of research into policy. It offers suggestions for the creative use of qualitative research designs and of qualitative narratives, in addition to traditional quantitative research designs, to improve and strengthen the relationship between both sides. It makes an argument for the combined use of both designs in a mixed methodology approach that allows for a more insightful interpretation of quantitative findings, and, at the same time, for a more broadly applicable substantiation of qualitative findings. Finally, it provides specific case examples of qualitative research, from informal to formal, that have successfully influenced policy and/or created systems change.

THE RELATIONSHIP BETWEEN RESEARCH AND POLICY

Today populations in developed Western societies are growing more diverse and older and they are facing more complex social and environmental stressors than ever before. Of primary concern continues to be the impact of social problems on physical and psychological health, and governments everywhere are aware of the need to address them more systemically through the development and implementation of creative policies and programs. Thus, they have begun to focus on re-structuring the funding, organization, and delivery of health services in their respective countries (Davis & Howden-Chapman, 1996). In the United States, legislators and policy makers now have a much greater and ever-changing need for up-to-date information in order to carry out their governmental responsibility for the development of responsive state health policy (Coburn, 1998).

Evidence is mounting for the advantages of considering research findings when making health-related decisions to ensure their viability and applicability (Anderson, Cosby, Swan, Moore, & Broekhoven, 1999; Sheldon, Guyatt, & Haines, 1998). Health researchers and policy makers tend to agree that combining the best efforts of each side will facilitate the provision of more effective health care in a practical manner. At the same time, blending research and practice will require additional efforts to integrate the significant differences between practitioners and researchers in their prior training, work and personal experience, and focus and philosophy (Carise et al., 2002).

MODELS OF THE RELATIONSHIP BETWEEN RESEARCH AND POLICY

Traditionally, discussions on how research and policy relate to each other have focused on delineating the various relationships that characterize how policy may flow from, or be affected by, research. In reviewing the extant literature (for example, Anderson et al., 1999; Black, 2001; Davis & Howden-Chapman, 1996; Trostle et al., 1999; Weiss, 1977), it is possible to define the relationships between research and policy according to a continuum with three points, including (1) the logical model, which views the connection between research and policy as highly structured and linear, with policy flowing directly from, and being impacted directly by, research; (2) the political model, which views the connection between research and policy as dependent upon the political arena, with research being purposefully and deliberately manipulated either to support or oppose predetermined policy positions; and (3) the conceptual model, which views the connection between research and policy as indirect and diffuse, recognizing that neither influences, and is influenced by, the other alone but that both emerge in the context of complex social processes.

While the logical model is seen today as idealistic and overly simplistic and the political model as disheartening and with cynicism, the conceptual model is generally accepted as most realistic. Researchers and policy makers are beginning to agree that they represent two groups among many that come together to pool their talents, beliefs, and understanding in an effort to make sense of a problem (Weiss, 1977). Doing so can help to negotiate the contrasting perspectives of different stakeholders as they engage in interactive discourse. It may lead to a change in thinking of various community organizations, as they are affected by and reflect upon the issue under investigation, and ultimately may change the community itself (Anderson et al., 1999). To be sure, such global re-orientation is unlikely to be spurred by one single research study alone. Rather, it is the gradual accumulation of complementary research that leads to far-reaching and enduring changes in the way people and their governments confront societal issues (Weiss, 1977) and that ultimately transforms society as a whole.

THE RESEARCH-TO-PRACTICE GAP

Much has been written about the potential reasons for the poor transfer of research, health-related and other, into policy and the resulting research-to-practice gap. These reasons can be more readily elucidated by contrasting health research with policy and practice in terms of specific training, work activities, and topical relevance. As Schor (2000) explains, health research is usually performed by highly educated individuals, while health practice is performed by people with great variability in training. Health research seeks to create new knowledge and guide relevant work by directly building on existing information, while health practice seeks to apply knowledge and often must develop policies and programs in the absence of necessary information. Finally, health research is primarily geared towards educating professionals, while health practice is geared towards educating the public. Simply put, health research is aimed at understanding the healthcare delivery system, while health policy is aimed at directing it (Rosenthal, 1981).

Issues of Specificity. Developing effective and relevant policy is a complex process that requires a great amount of contextual knowledge, including policy content, policy history, legislative procedures, key actors, and constituencies (Coburn, 1998). Health policy seeks to address problems that are the result of many composite forces located in a complex, yet uncertain, environment. Consequently, it faces the challenging task of taking into account contextual qualifications and environmental uncertainties in order to produce viable responses.

In fact, researchers are quite well accustomed to concentrating on complex issues and incorporating the myriad of conditional ambiguities that are part of the real-life research setting. However, as a rule, they interpret results in terms that are reflective of potential limitations and alternative explanations (Roos & Shapiro, 1999). In their work, they send messages often viewed as being "too complicated, irrelevant, 'ivory tower,' and therefore, not helpful" (Rosenthal, 1981, p. 13). Their findings are seen as too "scientific" and lacking the ability to clearly capture the concerns policy makers have. They often fail to produce what policy makers really want: a clear and straightforward endorsement of one policy alternative over another. Thus, their work ultimately loses its relevance. Policy makers, on the other hand, show a great predilection towards using information from peers, local and national experts, and other informal sources (Feldman et al., 2001). They may even base their decisions on tacit knowledge, personal experience, or anecdotes. In formulating the research question, researchers seldom consider its applicability and relevance to health policy. Their simplistic view of how policy is made and how research can impact on the policy protocol evidences political naiveté. They must face their work being ignored or having only an indirect impact on policy and learn to accept the independence of the political process (Black, 2001; Rozzini & Trabucchi, 2001).

Issues of Timeliness. In their quest to develop new and relevant knowledge, researchers often need a considerable amount of time to design and implement a scientifically sound research methodology and then analyze the data in an empirically rigorous manner. In addition, they customarily choose to disseminate their findings by publishing them in academic journals. The transformation of raw data into research results and, subsequently, into a final report, including manuscript preparation, submission, review, and publication is lengthy and typically lasts many months, even years. Unfortunately, results that are published long after a policy has been implemented, regardless of their accuracy and conclusiveness, no longer carry any real informative meaning for that policy. In fact, policy makers prefer preliminary but timely results over more definite but delayed results and are more likely to use them in their decision-making (Feldman et al., 2001). Researchers who are familiar enough with the dynamic nature of the policy process may be able to anticipate up-and-coming issues, allowing them sufficient lead time to plan and carry out relevant work within an adequate time frame (Merrill & Somers, 1985).

Clearly, making the policy process a priority requires a shift in thinking for most academic researchers. Although universities have historically emphasized a combined mission of teaching, research, and public service, the latter has been neglected relative to the former two. The low perceived value of public service is rooted in university criteria for faculty promotion and tenure, which continue to assign utmost significance to peer-reviewed journal publications (Coburn, 1998). Many faculty researchers perceive applied policy-related projects as too labor-intensive relative their potential for professional advancement. They are not yet willing to move beyond the passive reporting of research to its active dissemination and translation into policy (Davis & Howden-Chapman, 1996). Such an "intertwining of the research and policy roles and the infusion of political values into the heart of the research enterprise" (Fudge & Barrett, cited in Davis & Howden-Chapman, 1996, p. 869) must occur in order to more accurately reflect the true nature of the policy-making process as inherently unstructured and value-oriented.

Issues of Communication. Perhaps most significantly, the nature and quality of the communicative interactions that occur between researchers and policy makers are generally quite poor and lack common ground. In fact, researcher and policy makers do not even speak the same professional language, either in verbal or written communications (Feldman et al., 2001). For example, although researchers are well versed in preparing analytical and/or research reports, they find it difficult to "translate" these reports into language more readily understandable to policy makers. Theoretical terms such as "independent/dependent/confounding variable," "reliability/validity," and "selection bias" on the research side are juxtaposed with practical terms such as "Medicaid Waiver," "federal/state mandate," and "inter-agency contracts" on the policy side. Researchers are often unprepared or unwilling to share their findings directly with policy makers. Rather, they believe that publishing their results in scientific journals is sufficient to make them available to, and usable for, a broader audience (Trostle et al., 1999). Yet, with some ingenuity and only minor modifications, they can prepare reports of quantitative findings that are much more user-friendly and thus are much more likely to be used.

Policy makers have grown quite frustrated with this academic approach and express a desire for researchers to articulate the policy implications of findings more clearly. Moreover, they criticize reporting formats that comply with academic standards because such formats are often inappropriate for their purposes and show little direct policy-related relevance (Feldman et al., 2001). For example, omission of the executive summary and emphasis of textual over graphical content often precludes a "quick read." Consequently many policy makers simply do not bother with research published under these formats, resulting in a considerable amount of arguably important information presented in academic journals of which policy makers have never even heard (Merrill & Somers, 1985). As Roos and Shapiro (1999) suggest, if complex research reports are to be successfully communicated rather than to "gather dust" (p. JS298), they should be written like stories, for stories "stick in the mind better than statistics" (p. JS302). More broadly put, policy makers are much more likely to read, and pay attention to, material from which they can extract easily discernible, easily digestible, and visually pleasing information that is timely and applicable to the real-life problems affecting their constituencies.

Undoubtedly, the manner in which quantitative researchers, and to some extent qualitative researchers as well, have traditionally disseminated their findings has contributed to their poor translation into policy. In fact, the typical research report with its lack of clarity, intelligibility, and relevance to all but a very limited audience may well be one of the most significant barriers to the use of research by policy makers (Funk, Tornquist, & Champagne, 1995). Few researchers will question the notion that they write for an audience, and that audience may or may not share their assumptions or language (Belgrave, Zablotsky, & Guadagno, 2002; Creswell, 1998). But because it is the intent of the qualitative report to produce narrative description and/or analysis that is full and rich with detail, it has great potential for capturing and sustaining the attention of a broader audience. Traditional formats for communicating findings, which are primarily concerned with efficiency, provide only an imperfect route for the dissemination of qualitative research (Boyd & Munhall, 2001). As a general rule, qualitative reports present findings in formats that reflect the method of qualitative inquiry used in the study (Boyd & Munhall, 2001; Creswell, 1998; Wolcott, 2002), and as such, although they may not adhere to the reporting format commonly used for academic journals, they may be eminently more readable.

USING QUALITATIVE RESEARCH TO INFLUENCE POLICY

In recent years, researchers have become increasingly sensitive to the lack of attention paid to their work by policy makers. In seeking alternative methods to develop truly evocative definitions of human phenomena and explain them as they exist in the real world, they have become increasingly aware of the need to move beyond the traditional quantitative, or positivist, research paradigm. This approach generally incorporates standardized, self-administered or interviewer-administered surveys and/or questionnaires and large study samples and leads to analytic reports that overflow with numerical and statistical data and are largely ignored by policy makers. Because quantitative research is generally less concerned with the specificity, timeliness, and communication of findings than with their reliability, validity, and generalizability, it has traditionally done a poor job of capturing and conveying the full depth and breadth of the multitude of human experiences. It is for this reason that quantitative researchers have come to be viewed as detached and dispassionate experimenters who expend great effort on manipulating their subjects in various laboratory settings but spend little effort on implementing their results in various real-life settings.

On the other hand, the qualitative, or naturalistic, research paradigm allows for the unique perspectives of small groups of people to be explored in detail. A distinct strength of this approach is its power to "detect, represent, and explicate the meaning of something from the viewpoint of the actors involved" (Sankar & Gubrium, 1994, p. x). It thereby provides a rich description of phenomena that "opens a window into the world of others" (Morse & Field, 1995, p. 18) and leads to reports that foster better understanding of a phenomenon "as is," as it is present in the natural environment (Denzin, 1988). In fact, one of the hallmarks of qualitative research is its tradition of community-based fieldwork that invites more reflexive, pluralist, and interpretive modes of inquiry (Denzin & Lincoln, 1994). Increasingly, the role of the traditional researcher who remains distant and value free in the search for a single, objective truth, often at the expense of those who are "being researched," is being challenged to become more activist-oriented and open to true partnership and collaboration with, and empowerment of the communities on whose behalf research is being done (Fine, 1994; Wallerstein, 1999).

Activist-Oriented Models of Research. Today, the emphasis on objectivity and expertness, along with the separation of research from practice advocated by the positivist paradigm is shifting towards much greater participation of non-academic researchers in the process of creating knowledge (Israel, Schulz, Parker, & Becker, 1998). This shift from research done "on communities" to research done "with communities" has revived the old tradition of Kurt Lewin's action research from the 1940s (Wallerstein, 1999) and has given rise to a number of alternative research models that often combine quantitative and qualitative methods, variously called participatory action research, empowerment evaluation, feminist research, community-based/participatory/involved/collaborative/centered research (Israel et al., 1998). Participatory action research is not a distinct research design; rather, it is an approach to doing research that is based on an interactive collaboration between all stakeholders invested in a common social issue (Hammel, Finlayson, & Lastowski, 2003). All activist-oriented models of research are explicitly committed to participants shaping and leading the research design, assuming control of research processes, and benefiting from the research either through direct intervention or by using it to inform action for social systems change (Israel et al., 1998; Friedman, 2001; Minkler, 2004). These models actually facilitate systems change by providing a more authentic, contextual explanation of findings, often by inviting long-marginalized voices in the community to share their narratives and stories (Rappaport, 1995).

What follows below are three case examples of how qualitative research has been used to inform public policy and bring about systems change. The examples range from informal use to a mixed methods approach to formal application of qualitative techniques and from verbal communications to executive summary report to published dissemination of findings. It is this flexibility in choice of designs and dissemination channels that makes qualitative research such a good fit for policy change.

Case Example #1: Medicaid Advocacy. Using qualitative research to influence social policy does not necessarily require rigorous naturalistic inquiry and formally trained qualitative researchers. As an example, the Optional Coverage for Women and Infants (OCWI) Medicaid Advocacy Project highlights how qualitative techniques can be used informally yet creatively to inform social policy. It developed from efforts by a state agency in a Southeastern state to evaluate the state's Medicaid service system. Between 1991 and 2000, the agency ran a Medicaid Advocacy Hotline, staffed by volunteers who handed calls from pregnant women, mothers of young children, and other family members from across the state. Volunteers collected demographic and other quantitative data and documented numerous problems with and/or access barriers to the existing service system. Hotline information was also used to create thousands of "advocacy summaries," shown in Figure 1, brief narratives of 3 to 8 sentences, compiled by county and by month/year that gave a qualitative description of the personal experiences of callers with the system.

The advocacy summaries were shared on a monthly basis with a statewide interagency maternal and child health "Access Task Force," which explored themes of problems in particular agencies or counties further. In 1994, due to proposed legislative budget cuts, the OCWI program under Medicaid was greatly endangered. To demonstrate to state legislators the need for continuing the program, the state agency pro-

FIGURE 1. Case Example #1: Sample Advocacy Summaries

Sample 1	*Father of a 23-year-old pregnant woman called for assistance arranging an appointment for Medicaid application for daughter. She was staying in a domestic violence shelter for her protection from abusive husband. She had to leave her car and belongings when she fled; thus, transportation is a problem. After she did get transportation, she reported to Department of Social Services (DSS) on the weekday instructed by DSS but was told that OCWI applications are only taken between 8:00 a.m. and 10:30 a.m., and that only 7 applications are taken per day (she had arrived at 11:00 a.m.)*
Sample 2	*A 30-year-old female with 1-ms baby called for assistance with an OCWI Medicaid problem. She had gone to DSS in August to apply only for OCWI to cover her pregnancy. Confused, she ended up applying for Aid to Families with Dependent Children (AFDC). She was denied AFDC 5 months later because one of her children's social security numbers was a duplicate number. DSS worker did not refer her for OCWI Medicaid for her pregnancy (and now baby) even though she knew the woman came in specifically for Medicaid, had no health insurance, and had no way to pay for health care. The AFDC case went on for several months before the woman was denied, while she believed she was under consideration for Medicaid the entire time.*

vided them with advocacy summaries from their constituent areas along with quantitative data regarding the success of the OCWI program. Based on these narrative accounts, legislators were able to see firsthand the "impossible situations" families in poverty were experiencing, and the OCWI program was ultimately spared.

Case Example #2: Service Linkage for People with Traumatic Brain Injury. This case example illustrates how qualitative techniques can be creatively incorporated into a formal quantitative research design to augment and enhance an otherwise wholly statistical analysis and to infuse findings with a "human element." The Traumatic Brain Injury Service Linkage project was developed and conducted in 2001 as complement to a larger study, the Traumatic Brain Injury Registry and Follow-Up System (TBIRFS) study, a collaborative effort between several state agencies and universities in a Southeastern state. The study was designed to evaluate the existing service system for persons with TBI and their family members in the state and to assess the effectiveness of a follow-up registry that tracked these persons over time. It relied on the qualitative tool of focus group discussions to aid in the in-depth exploration of the unique experience of living with TBI and of the unique service needs due to TBI through consumer stories. The rationale for the use of focus groups rests on the theoretical tenet that people develop attitudes and perceptions not in isolation but through interaction with others (Morse & Field, 1995).

A descriptive analysis of conversations from the focus groups, four in all, showed that persons with TBI and their family members living in the Southeastern state under study identified five common needs in reference to the existing service system. As shown in Figure 2, each need was ultimately identified by reviewing, sorting, condensing actual "raw" language statements into groups of conceptual themes and then into categories of common needs.

In all, five categories were identified, reflecting the need for (1) an early, consistent and comprehensive service system; (2) information and education; (3) formal and informal advocacy; (4) resourcefulness in and empowerment of persons with TBI and their families; and (5) human connectedness and social belonging (for a more detailed discussion of the project and its results, see Leith, Phillips, & Sample, 2004). The descriptive analysis regarding the lived experiences and service needs of people with TBI and their family members were shared with key stakeholders in the project, including the state's Brain Injury Alliance (BIA) group, who used findings of the five categories of common needs to educate state legislators about TBI. Ultimately, the group was suc-

FIGURE 2. Case Example #2: Illustration of Need Identificatiòn

Natural Language Statement →	Conceptual Theme →	Category of Common Need
"We need something like home-bound care. Like when the nurses go out and help. Assistance . . . any-body . . .even if it's just for a little while." *"Just having . . . if somebody just came out to the house two to three times a week. . ."*	To offer comprehen-sive home health care services, particularly informal services.	Need for early, consistent, comprehensive service system.
"It was tough. We wandered aimlessly for a long time!" *"I don't think there's much for the family, or the wife, or the sister, or the person that's going to have to do stuff."*	To consider creation of a state-wide agency responsible for a comprehensive TBI service delivery system.	

cessful in pursuing legislation that created a state brain injury fund from fines levied against aggressive drivers. Another stakeholder, the state's Department of Vocational Rehabilitation increased specialized brain injury training for staff and is developing a pilot Brain Injury Program. And finally, several of the focus group participants were empowered by their conversations with their peers and by the connections they were able to form in the focus groups and have since become more involved in BIA and related TBI advisory council efforts.

Case Example #3: Family Caregiver Support Program Evaluation. Of course, as time and financial resources permit, qualitative research may seek to inform public policy through formal naturalistic inquiry, coupled with reflective analysis rather than analytic description, as evidenced by the third case example. This project, the Family Caregiver Support Program (FCSP) evaluation, is initiated annually by the Southeastern state agency charged with administering the FCSP. The agency collaborated with researchers to focus the 2004 evaluation on assessing the process of implementation of the program as well as the program's impact and effectiveness in achieving its intended goals during the evaluation period. The evaluation incorporated both a qualitative and a quantitative measurement component. The qualitative component involved activities that provided in-depth, unstructured, non-numerical data to monitor/assess the basic service elements of the project by identifying service activities and how they were delivered; the types of barriers and opportunities that affected how well activities were achieved; and the types of individual, organizational, and systems characteristics that affected how well they were achieved.

Qualitative activities consisted of the formal collection and analysis of data through (1) in-depth, face-to-face interviews with twelve service providers, asking them to share their thoughts, ideas, and opinions about the program, perceived areas of success or lack thereof, progress or lack thereof towards established goals, and perceived structural/procedural barriers/opportunities to successful program maintenance; and (2) focus group discussions, three in all, with (a) service consumers, asking them to share their thoughts and opinions regarding benefits of the program to the care-giving experience, potential gaps in the program, and overall impact of the program on their lives; and (b) service administrators, asking them to share their feedback regarding structural and organizational aspects of the program, barriers and facilitators to its continued implementation, and continued sustainability of the program over time.

Formal qualitative data analysis involved the process of identifying, coding, and categorizing patterns and themes and then reducing the number of categories by selecting, ordering, and clustering them. After initial manual coding of the information, it was transferred into a computer software program specifically designed for qualitative data analysis for further content analysis, an analysis by topic segmented into categories. As shown in Figure 3, the final product was a theme "codebook," a hierarchy of common, overarching themes synthesized across all qualitative data that reflected a theoretical understanding of service provider, service consumer, and service administrator perceptions regarding the effectiveness of the FCSP.

Final results of both the qualitative and the quantitative analyses were shared with the state agency in the form of a narrative report that explicated the findings by providing actual quotes of study participants. The findings ultimately led to a change in the way the state agency trains

FIGURE 3. Case Example #3: Illustration of Formal Theme Hierarchy

	Theme Structure	*Main Theme and Related Sub-Themes*
1	**1**	***FLEXIBILITY MAKES* the Family Caregiver Support Program**
2	1.1	Flexibility does span all levels
3	1.2	Flexibility differs in importance across levels
4	1.3	Flexibility means creative interpretation of guidelines
5	1.4	Flexibility should be balanced with uniformity
6	**2**	**The *ADVOCATE IS* the Family Caregiver Support Program**
7	2.1	Advocates love what they do
8	2.2	The advocate's job is never done
9	2.3	Advocate strengths & weaknesses shape the program
10	2.4	Advocate training is key
11	**3**	**The *CAREGIVER OWNS* the Family Caregiver Support Program**
12	3.1	Caregivers value the program greatly
13	3.2	Caregivers value consumer choice moderately
14	3.3	Caregivers do not fully recognize the program's aims/limitations
15	**4**	***COMMITMENT SUSTAINS* the Family Caregiver Support Program**
16	4.1	Commitment means willingness to give . . . financially and collaboratively
17	4.2	Commitment must span all levels
18	4.3	Commitment means evolving the program not maintaining it

its FCSP service providers upon initial hiring and contributed to a re-focusing of program goals away from predominantly financial assistance and towards consumer education and training. In addition, they highlighted the need for the development of more formal outcomes measures by which to assess the FCSP in the future. As a result, efforts are currently underway to (1) define more specifically what outcomes should be measured and how to measure them; and (2) design a data entry system capable of capturing the selected outcomes.

CONCLUSION

Despite the persistent and often frustrating difficulties researchers and policy makers encounter in their mutual interactions, both sides agree that health research can, and does, make valuable contributions to the development of relevant health policy. Thus the question no longer is whether health research should be used at all, but how it can be used more effectively to inform health policy (Rosenthal, 1981). In the search for answers, efforts are underway at local, state, even federal governmental agencies and university research departments alike to learn more about the exigencies each side faces and to find a common basis for interaction. As Coburn (1998) indicates, although relationships between states and their universities vary in formality and quality, strategic alliances between the two are becoming increasingly commonplace. The push towards action-oriented models of research, including participatory action research and community-based participatory research, has been prompted in part because of community demands for greater involvement and in part because of government and private funder mandates for coalitions, community advisory boards, and community engagement (see Wallerstein, 1999). Indeed, the recent Request for Applications RFA-MD-05-002, National Center on Minority Health and Health Disparities Community Participation in Health Disparities Intervention Research, issued by the National Institutes of Health (National Institutes of Health, 2005) highlights the increasing recognition of the importance for innovative research that is jointly conducted by communities and researchers. It also shows growing enthusiasm on all sides for developing cross-cutting strategies and guidelines that can help to foster more effective exchanges between the research and practice fields.

As shown in the preceding discussion, the emergence of qualitative research in addition to more traditional study methods, ranging from the informal use of qualitative techniques to a fully-developed naturalistic design, has the potential to greatly enhance the relationship between research and policy and aid in the more efficient translation of research findings into public policy. This relationship can become truly satisfying only if researchers and policy makers are willing to negotiate the language and the frame of reference even before research is initiated (Davis & Howden-Chapman, 1996). Researchers may indeed be guilty of "academizing" their work, gearing it predominately towards their peers and making it difficult for non-academicians to read and understand their reports. Communication and dissemination of qualitative research findings prefers modes that include narratives, case studies, and personal stories related to people's experiences with and thoughts and opinions about social problems. Reports incorporating these modes of writing are much more likely to be read by and be useful to policy makers. Thus, researchers who truly seek to influence policy should seriously consider research designs that incorporate a strong qualitative component.

REFERENCES

Anderson, M., Cosby, J., Swan, B., Moore, H., & Broekhoven, M. (1999). The use of research in local health service agencies. *Social Science and Medicine*, *49*(8), 1007-19.

Belgrave, L. L., Zablotsky, D., & Guadagno, M. A. (2002). How do we talk to each other? Writing qualitative research for quantitative researchers. *Qualitative Health Research*, *12*(10), 1427-1439.

Black, N. (2001). Evidence based policy: Proceed with care. *British Medical Journal*, *323*, 275-9.

Boyd, C. O., & Munhall, P. L. (2001). Qualitative research proposals and reports. In P. L. Munhall (Ed.), *Nursing research: A qualitative perspective* (3rd ed.) (pp. 613-638). Sudbury, MA: Jones & Bartlett.

Carise, D., Cornely, W., & Gurel, O. (2002). A successful researcher-practitioner collaboration in substance abuse treatment. *Journal of Substance Abuse Treatment*, *23*(2), 157-62.

Coburn, A. F. (1998). The role of health services research in developing state health policy. *Health Affairs*, *17*(1), 139-51.

Creswell, J. W. (1998). *Qualitative inquiry and research design: Choosing among five traditions*. Thousand Oaks, CA: Sage.

Davis, P., & Howden-Chapman, P. (1996). Section T: Translating research findings into health policy. *Social Science and Medicine*, *43*(5), 865-72.

Denzin, N. K. (1988). *Interpretive interactionism*. Newbury Park, CA: Sage.

Denzin, N. K., & Lincoln, Y. S. (1994). Introduction: Entering the field of qualitative research. In N. K. Denzin & Y. S. Lincoln (Eds.), *Handbook of qualitative research* (pp. 1-17). Thousand Oaks, CA: Sage.

Feldman, P. H., Nadash, P., & Gursen, M. (2001). Improving communications between researchers and policy makers in long-term care: Or, researchers are from Mars: Policy makers are from Venus. *The Gerontologist*, *41*(3), 312-21.

Fine, M. (1994). Working the hyphens: Reinventing self and other in qualitative research. In: N. K. Denzin & Y. S. Lincoln (Eds.), *Handbook of qualitative research* (pp. 70-82). Thousand Oaks, CA: Sage.

Friedman, V. 92001). Action science: Creating communities of inquiry in communities of practice. In P. Reason & H. Bradbury (Eds.), *Handbook of action research: Participatory inquiry and practice* (pp. 159-171). Thousand Oaks, CA: Sage.

Funk, S. G., Tornquist, E. M., & Champagne, M. T. (1995). Barriers and facilitators of research utilization. *Nursing Clinics of North America*, *30*(3), 395-407.

Institute of Medicine. (1998). *Bridging the gap between practice and research: Forging partnerships with community-based drug and alcohol treatment*. Washington, DC: National Academy of Sciences Press.

Israel, B. A., Schulz, A. J., Parker, E. A., & Becker, A. B. (1998). Review of community-based research: Assessing partnership approaches to improve public health. *Annual Review of Public Health*, *19*, 173-202.

Leith, K. H., Phillips, L., & Sample, P. L. (2004). Exploring the service needs of persons with TBI and their families: The South Carolina experience. *Brain Injury*, *18*(12), 1191-1208.

Merrill, J. C., & Somers, S. A. (1985). Does health services research affect public policy? *Health Span, 2*(5), 18-21.

Minkler, M. (2004). Ethical challenges for the "outside" researcher in community-based participatory research. *Health Education and Behavior, 31*(6), 684-697.

Morse, J. M., & Field, P. A. (1995). *Qualitative research methods for health professionals* (2nd Ed.). Sage Publications: Thousand Oaks.

National Institutes of Health. (2005). NCMHD Community Participation in Health Disparities Intervention Research. RFA-MD-05-002. Retrieved March 1, 2005, from http://grants1.nih.gov/grants/guide/rfa-files/RFA-MD-05-002.html.

Rappaport, J. (1995). Empowerment meets narrative: Listening to stories and creating settings. *American Journal of Community Psychology, 23*(5), 795-806.

Roos, N. P., & Shapiro, E. (1999). From research to policy: What have we learned? *Medical Care, 37*(6), JS291-JS305.

Rosenthal, G. (1981). Does good health services research produce good health policy? *Health Policy Quarterly, 1*(1), 8-21.

Rozzini, R., & Trabucchi, M. (2001). To the editor. *The Gerontologist, 41*(6), 830-1.

Sandelowski, M. (1998). Writing a good read: Strategies for re-presenting qualitative data. *Research in Nursing and Health, 21*, 375-382.

Sankar, A., & Gubrium, J. F. (1994). Introduction. In J. F. Gubrium & A. Sankar (Eds.), *Qualitative methods in aging research* (pp. vii-xvii). Thousand Oaks, CA: Sage.

Schor, E. (2000). *Conference summary: Building bridges for child health research, policy and practice*. Retrieved September 17, 2004, from www.ahcpr.gov/research/bridgesch/bridge2.htm.

Sheldon, T. A., Guyatt, G. H., & Haines, A. (1998). Getting research findings into practice: When to act on evidence. *British Medical Journal, 317*, 139-42.

Trostle, J., Bronfman, M., & Langer, A. (1999). How do researchers influence decision-makers: Case studies of Mexican policies. *Health Policy and Planning, 14*(2), 103-14.

Wallerstein, N. (1999). Power between evaluator and community: Research relationships within New Mexico's healthier communities. *Social Science and Medicine, 49*(1), 39-53.

Weiss, C. H. (1977). *Using social research in public policy making*. Lexington, MA: Lexington Books.

Wolcott, H. F. (2002). Writing up qualitative research . . . better. *Qualitative Health Research, 12*(1), 91-103.

Quality of Life in Nursing Homes: Involving Elders in Policy Making for Their Own Care and Life Satisfaction

Kathryn McKinley
Geri Adler

SUMMARY. The Nursing Home Reform Act (NHRA) of 1987 established nursing home requirements and dually emphasized quality of care and quality of life outcomes. We researched elders' perceptions of quality of life in nursing homes using focus groups. Analysis revealed four major themes important to residents: generativity, spiritual well-being, homelike environment, and privacy. Themes were used to analyze the disparity between NHRA's goal of dual emphasis and the dominance of quality of care in the treatment of frail elders living in nursing homes. Policies and procedures must be developed that promote decisional control in everyday matters of an older person's life.

KEYWORDS. Nursing homes, elderly, quality of life

Kathryn McKinley, MSW, is affiliated with the Social Work Department, Buena Vista University, 610 West 4th Street, Storm Lake, IA 50588 (E-mail: McKinley@bvu.edu).

Geri Adler, MSW, PhD, is affiliated with the College of Social Work, University of South Carolina, Columbia, SC 29208 (E-mail: geri.adler@sc.edu).

[Haworth co-indexing entry note]: "Quality of Life in Nursing Homes: Involving Elders in Policy Making for Their Own Care and Life Satisfaction." McKinley, Kathryn, and Geri Adler. Co-published simultaneously in *The Social Policy Journal* (The Haworth Press, Inc.) Vol. 4, No. 3/4, 2005, pp. 37-51; and: *Cutting-Edge Social Policy Research* (ed: Richard Hoefer) The Haworth Press, Inc., 2005, pp. 37-51. Single or multiple copies of this article are available for a fee from The Haworth Document Delivery Service [1-800-HAWORTH, 9:00 a.m. - 5:00 p.m. (EST). E-mail address: docdelivery@haworthpress.com].

Available online at http://www.haworthpress.com/web/SPJ

doi:10.1300/J185v04n03_03

INTRODUCTION

Since passage of the Nursing Home Reform Act (NHRA) as part of the Omnibus Budget Reconciliation Act of 1987, a dual emphasis has been placed on the quality of care and the quality of life of long-term care residents (Arcus, 1999; Chapin & Cox, 2001). While long-term care can be provided in many settings, nursing homes most frequently come to mind as providing care for the frail elderly.

Over 1.7 million adults reside in nursing homes (U.S. Census Bureau, 2000). Most residents are elderly (Atchely & Barusch, 2004), female, white, and in need of assistance with activities of daily living (Hooyman & Kiyak, 2002). Nursing homes are considered to be the most restrictive housing alternative along the long-term care continuum (Atchley & Barusch, 2004), governed by rigid routines and regulations that promote institutional efficiency and resident dependency (Kane, Caplan, Urv-Wong, Freeman, Aroskar, & Finch, 1997). There is a greater supply of nursing home beds and fewer long-term care options in rural America; thus the rates of institutionalization are higher than in urban areas (National Rural Health Association, 2001).

The NHRA led to changes in the way care is provided within the long-term care industry, tightening survey and certification procedures, mandating staff training, introducing social work services, and reducing the use of physical and chemical restraints (Zhang & Grabowski, 2004). While quality of life and quality of care were presented as equally important to the provision of care, several analyses have shown that the NHRA has fallen short of its goals (Harrington, 2002; Hillier & Barrow, 1999; Report to Congress, 2001; Wunderlich & Kohler, 2001).

Some (Cox, 1993; Cruikshank, 2003; Kane & Kane, 2001) consider the attitudes toward elderly nursing home residents paternalistic. Because residents are some of the oldest and most frail members of society, it is assumed they are unable to make decisions and choices in their own interest. Family members are often asked questions about expectations for daily life and staff makes decisions based on nursing home policy, accreditation standards, and other regulations. Consequently, residents become less sure of their own abilities and learn to become increasingly helpless (Cox, 1993; Harvey, 2001).

A nursing home is foremost a resident's "home," yet research has shown that they have little to say about everyday choices of what to eat, when to get up in the morning, or with whom to spend their time (Kane et al., 1997; Ouslander, 1995). Space for personal belongings is scarce. Privacy is rare. For rural elders, who have fewer housing choices than their urban counterparts, these concerns are especially cogent. Within the parameters of regulation, it is the nursing home's responsibility to foster resident autonomy and individuation. It is our belief that to advance the quality of life and achieve the outcomes that elderly nursing home residents desire, they must identify, prioritize, and frame their own needs. The objectives of this research study are to examine rural older nursing home residents' perceptions of their ability to participate in decision-making at the facilities in which they reside as well the activities, behaviors, and opportunities that facilitate their quality of life. We conducted a series of focus groups to gain understanding of rural resident perceptions of quality of life issues. These perceptions were used to critique the NHRA mandate for a service framework that emphasizes quality of life.

THEORETICAL FRAMEWORK

Lynott and Lynott (1996) claim that theory was nearly absent from gerontological research prior to 1961. No current theory adequately explains the experience of older adults in nursing homes. However, client-centered theory and ageism may help frame the issue and begin to develop a model for understanding policy and practice with older adults in nursing homes.

At its core, resident-centered care is about quality of life. It embodies the concept of self-determination, a foundation for social work practice. Client-centered theory, and the resultant resident-focused care are based on the assumption that residents know what matters to them, and, if provided the opportunities to do so, are capable of directing their environment (Turner, 1986; MMRC, 2002). The participants in our study enacted this theory. They expressed their personal life preferences and, when given the chance, had ideas about priorities for their facilities. They found creative ways to make meaning for their lives even within the confines of personal and environmental restrictions.

Ageism provides a model by which to understand quality of life issues in nursing homes. By definition, ageism is the "process of systematic stereotyping and discrimination against people because they are old" (Butler, 1987, p. 22). It portrays the ageing process as inescapable decline whereby older adults become isolated, in poor health, unable to be productive, and inevitably institutionalized (Kart & Kinney, 2001). Such assumptions color how society and, in particular, facilities and helping professionals, treat and care for the old.

The policies and procedures that direct the care provided in nursing homes largely mirror the attitudes and beliefs held by society toward the old. For example, ageist attitudes can be seen in the different approaches taken toward caring for younger nursing home residents. According to Kane and Kane (2001), a strong effort has been made to normalize the setting for younger people with disabilities who reside in nursing homes. An emphasis has been placed on consumer-direction whereby younger residents have increased control of staffing and daily routine. At such facilities, individualized accommodations are expected in the least restrictive environment (Chapin & Cox, 2001). In contrast, the choices available to elderly nursing home residents have remained limited with a continuing emphasis on protection and safety rather than decision-making and control. Ageist assumptions must be explicitly rejected in order for resident-centered care to succeed.

THE NURSING HOME REFORM ACT

The NHRA was the first major revision of Medicare and Medicaid standards for long term care since these programs were first created in 1965 (Turnham, n.d.). Public outcry over poor quality care in too many nursing homes led Congress to authorize an Institute of Medicine study of nursing home regulation (Turnham, n.d.). This report led to a new set of regulations known as the NHRA that was part of the Omnibus Reconciliation Act of 1987. These directives had widespread support by all significant stakeholder groups (Hawes, 1997).

Quality of Care

NHRA created federal minimum standards for the care and rights of people living in certified nursing facilities (Turnham, n.d.). Resident rights and quality of life received equal rank with quality of care (Hawes, 1997). Quality of care focused on providing the care and services needed to attain or maintain physical, mental, and psycho-social well-being. Activities of daily living (ADLs) were emphasized along with other physical needs. Mental and psycho-social functioning received brief mention as did the prevention of accidents, unnecessary drug use, and medication errors. Staff training and uniform facility standards were also included (Code of Federal Regulations, 42CFR483.25, 2003; Turnham, n.d.).

Quality of Life

While quality of care focused on the physical aspects of treatment that residents receive, quality of life centers on dignity, self-determination, and participation in social activities. Rights viewed as part of quality of life include being able to remain in the nursing home (barring certain conditions), the right to maintain or bank personal funds, return to the nursing home after hospitalizations or family visits, and review one's own medical records. Individualized care plans developed with the resident reflect self-determination. Reasonable accommodation of individual needs and preferences includes choice of personal physician. The right to participation refers to various activities as well as resident and family councils. Other areas included in quality of life are the provision of social services and a "safe, clean, comfortable, and homelike environment, allowing the resident to use his or her personal belongings to the extent possible" (Code of Federal Regulations, 42CFR483.15, 2003).

In 1999, the Health Care Financing Administration (HCFA) developed new regulations to strengthen federal oversight of nursing homes (Report to Congress, 2001). While improvement of quality of care was emphasized, there was no mention of quality of life issues. In 2001, Health and Human Services (HHS) released a study that addressed nurse staffing ratios in nursing homes (Report to Congress, 2001). This study also focused on quality of care and made no reference to quality of life. Zhang and Grabowski (2004) examined the effect of the NHRA on staffing and quality of care and concluded that while staffing is necessary to improved quality of care, it is not sufficient. The lack of attention to quality of life in the NHRA and the paucity of research on frail rural elders led us to wonder how this population viewed the issue of quality of life.

METHODS

Procedure

After obtaining institutional approval of the project, participants were recruited from nursing homes in three northwest Iowa rural communities to participate in focus groups. Community sizes ranged from under 1,000 to 10,000. The nursing homes averaged 72 beds, with the range being 66 to 89 beds. All nursing homes were non-profit and church related. Each had a social worker. All facilities described themselves as offering resident-centered care, a social model of care based on client-centered theory (Turner, 1986). It provides an individualized approach to meeting the emotional, physical, and spiritual needs and preferences of residents. Nursing homes implementing this approach emphasize self-determination, creativity, and teamwork. One facility in our study defines it "as a way of focusing the care delivery system on personal needs of the resident. It is centered on the pattern of life the resident had before entering [the facility]" (Methodist Manor Retirement Community [MMRC], 2002). A commitment to resident-centered care is expected to enhance the quality of the life of nursing home residents.

To be included in the study, subjects were required to be at least 65 years old, physically and cognitively able to participate in a focus group, and living in the facility at least six months. The six month criterion was selected because we were interested in only those for whom living at the nursing home was expected to be long term.

Participants

A total of 21 nursing home residents took part in four focus groups. There were 15 women and seven men. Their ages ranged from 80- to 101-years-old, with a mean age of 88.8 years. All participants were Euro-American which reflected the communities in which they lived. All residents needed assistance with at least two activities of daily living (ADLs). Participants had lived in the facilities from 6 months to 14 years.

Data Collection

Open-ended questions were explored with nursing home residents in four focus groups with four to seven participants. Focus groups enabled a reasonable size sample of residents to be interviewed while providing the opportunity for discussion and collaborative information sharing. All of the interviews followed a similar format and were audio-taped.

Each group interview lasted about one hour. A moderator began each group by explaining the purpose of the project and followed with an open-ended question asking residents what they believed contributed to their quality of life and satisfaction in the nursing home. The moderator continued using a predetermined list of prompts, which included general questions about decision-making, activities, physical space concerns, and interactions with other residents and staff. The moderator cued verbal exchanges throughout the discussion to keep it focused and made efforts to involve all participants. In addition, residents were asked their ages and reason for living in the nursing home. Race/ethnicity was observed as was gender.

The protocol was revised after each group to reflect themes that had emerged in the previous group. For example, if a new issue arose in a group discussion, a question related to that issue was added to the interview protocol.

Data Analysis

Interviews were transcribed verbatim including pauses, false starts, laughs, and other remarks. Each investigator reviewed the transcripts independently. On the first pass through the data, observations and impressions were coded, listed, and sorted into categories. Multiple readings of the transcripts and numerous discussions yielded compatible themes that clustered together and allowed us to organize key concepts. Four major themes were identified: generativity, spiritual well-being, homelike environment and privacy. These items are discussed in the following sections.

FINDINGS

Generativity

Generativity or caring and showing concern for others may be an important behavioral motivation for elderly nursing home residents (Erikson, Erickson, & Kivnik, 1986). Focus group participants reported a sense of fulfillment and purpose in behaviors that benefited others. For example, one female resident described herself as a "doer," mending items that other residents needed fixing while another sharpened pencils for staff.

A seminal generative act may be the actions residents show toward the dying in their institutions. With reverence and poignancy, residents spoke of their concern for the dying and their families. One noted that as her roommate was dying, "I gave up my room. I stayed out all the time that she was sick because they should . . . [her] three to four girls were always with her which I was so proud to think they could be with their mother." Another willingly gave of herself and her room as her, ". . . roommate passed away, some days got long and they were quite a . . . lovely family, . . . I just felt that the room should have been for them. And not me." Residents give of themselves, sometimes to inconvenience, to facilitate a private and personal experience for families as their relative died.

Spiritual Well-Being

Spirituality was an important dimension of well-being for the residents in our focus groups. Residents spoke of both personal spiritual experiences as well as religiosity. While both are powerful influences and multi-dimensional concepts, spirituality and religion cannot be used interchangeably. As explained by McInnis-Dittrich (2002), spirituality is "about finding meaning in life now and cultivating ways to explore and express those beliefs" (p. 267). Religion is a term used to describe a more formalized system of attitudes, beliefs, and practices. Persons can be spiritual but uninterested in attending organized religious services or even be anti-religious.

Residents described both spiritual and religious experiences. One lifelong farmer described the beauty of watching crops grow. She spoke almost mystically about being driven by nursing home staff to "look at the crops." The sheer joy and pleasure that emanated from that experience was palpable and a profoundly spiritual experience.

Others described their satisfaction with participation in church services. While church and synagogue attendance is higher for older adults than younger age groups (Hooyman & Kiyak, 2002), religious denomination was of little importance to our focus group participants. As noted by an 80-year-old female resident, "they have different church services. Catholic, Presbyterian, I'm not too churchy but Sunday." It is possible that for elders at this stage of their lives, religious belief and faith supercedes the more organizational aspects of religion (Hillier & Barrow, 1999). Elderly nursing home residents face many losses and challenges in everyday life. Spirituality and religion can help bring meaning and comfort to their lives (McInnis-Dittrich, 2002).

Homelike Environment

Most facilities describe themselves as the resident's home. They are resident-centered and interested in quality of life, yet most facilities do not resemble home. The concept of homelike, simple as it is, resonated with virtually all of the participants of this study. [You] "go to bed when you feel like it. It's important," stated a resident of one home while a person who lived in another stated "at home you're pretty independent. Here, pretty much we're told–you do what they tell you."

Harvey (2001) wonders why many nursing homes resemble hospitals, given that old age is a developmental stage. Indeed, the residents that were interviewed wondered very much the same thing. "The all-white, all-the-time, looks like a hospital." Another resident talked about the need for the dining room to be decorated. "But here what do we look at?–just those old bare walls. And it's not inviting."

Food is another area that residents relate to the concept of homelike. "The best meal is breakfast. It's homelike. Well, any breakfast food you want. You get orange juice and you get coffee and you get eggs and the rest of it [other meals] comes in tin cans." "Yesterday I said 'you know, I would like some cottage cheese and a fried egg.' I said I'm just craving a fried egg. And it wasn't exactly fried but it was something like that. Anyway I enjoyed it." Mok and Mui (1996) address empowerment of older adults living in nursing homes. This can often mean something as simple as being able to make one's own decisions. "To come and go as you please. To make your own decisions. To please yourself–you know." "Oh, if I want to go out, walk out, go to the sidewalk outdoors. If I want to take a time to go home, I go home. And if I want to skip a meal, I skip a meal. Kind of like you do at home."

These examples demonstrate that residents are not asking for extreme or dangerous items and activities but rather the right to a quality of life that most people take for granted. Frail elders living in rural nursing homes are simply dreaming of ways to recreate the lives that they used to lead when they could make decisions about the color of the walls, whether to walk outside, or what to eat for breakfast.

Privacy

Privacy is difficult to protect in a nursing home. Residents share rooms. Staff members often enter their rooms without warning or authorization. Public spaces are frequently crowded. It is no wonder that residents place a high value on privacy and that it needs to be addressed separately from the desire for a homelike environment (Harvey, 2001). One resident expressed this by saying "I would love to be by myself. It would make me feel at home. I could put my things where I want them around the room and be home." It is such a simple pleasure to be able to place objects where one wishes, and yet, most nursing home residents cannot do so.

Privacy also relates to social interaction. While maintaining social relationships is highly valued in society, this is not always available to nursing home residents. [I] "dropped out of two clubs because I didn't have room to entertain." In addition to space, residents talked about the lack of privacy when one cannot afford a private telephone or is no longer able to write her own letters.

Privacy relates to human dignity as expressed by the resident who said "They walk out and leave them (doors) wide open. I don't want them to see me when I have to lay down because I have a back ache."

And finally, privacy relates to generativity. Residents expressed conflict between wanting to help others and meet their own needs. "I'd like a private room. Where you have TV going most of the time, you have telephone calls, you can't have your conversation and try to help people [roommate] who can't pull blinds back and forth."

POLICY ANALYSIS

Changes Brought by NHRA

While the NHRA has led to numerous improvements, quality of care issues have continued to take precedence over quality of life issues (Hawes, 1997). For example, use of physical restraints and catheter use were decreased, and positive care practices such as activity involvement increased (Hawes et al., 1997; Kane, Williams, Williams, & Kane, 1993; Teno et al., 1997). Furthermore, residents achieved greater stability and slower rates of decline in ADLs, cognition and continence (Phillips et al., 1997).

The Impact of Ageism and Resident-Focused Care on Policy

Older adults living in nursing homes are the last residential population for which quality of life issues are being recognized. While ageism has been used to explain this situation, studies indicate that structures are as often the cause of ageism as individual bias (Gatz & Pearson, 1988; Robb, Chen, & Haley, 2002). Policy needs to focus on these structural issues and combine the theoretical with the practical when it comes to resident-focused care. Essential structures include (1) training of staff, (2) adequate staffing, (3) fiscal issues, (4) regulatory barriers, and (5) turf guarding (Hagebak & Hagebak, 1983; Robb, Chen, & Haley, 2002).

Several studies (Intrieri, Kelly, Brown, & Castilla, 1993; Hinrichsen & McMeniman, 2002; Hillman, Stricker, & Zweig, 1997) found that professionals' attitudes toward older adults became less negative with training. Staff need to be educated to approach residents from the perspective of "what does the resident want and how would she like to do it" rather than "what is good for the resident." Our participats emphasized that there needs to be staff on all shifts and those who work on weekends rather than just the weekday daytime shift. They also stressed that the education needs to include everyone from directors to maintenance staff. The NHRA provides the basis for this policy with its emphasis on quality of life.

A corollary to staff training is providing adequate staffing. Residents varied in how understanding they were of the nursing home being short-staffed but were in complete agreement that there were not enough staff to meet their needs. No matter how much employees want to focus on resident preferences, insufficient staff results in a focus on basic physical care that is provided within the confines of staff time rather than resident requests. Institutions may want to provide resident-focused care but lack the finances needed for adequate staff or training for their staff. State and federal policy needs to support financing that allows nursing homes to hire and train adequate staff. Some facilities have experimented with cross training staff to fill more than one position when needed.

Fiscal issues include both individual and institutional financial barriers (Gatz & Pearson, 1988). Participants who had spent their life savings on a year or two of care resented being denied privacy and consideration when they could no longer afford a private phone or day-to-day amenities such as choice of snacks or gifts for their grandchildren. They also had strong feelings about what the nursing homes should and should not spend money on. Carpet that made it difficult to maneuver wheelchairs was seen as a poor choice while air conditioning was seen as needed. Resident councils should be supported in efforts to provide input into decision making for the nursing home as well as for resident issues.

Regulatory barriers need to be reviewed in a holistic way. Nursing homes are regulated by multiple organizations whose standards frequently conflict. State and federal regulatory bodies need to review their policies with quality of life as a guiding principle. Agencies must also come to the table and review regulations together to reduce conflicts which serve to reduce quality of life. This. of course, brings up turf issues. Pressure must be brought to bear on agencies to focus on the quality of life of older adults rather than their own agency power. Those that cooperate with each other to do this should be rewarded.

The residents in our focus groups valued both quality of life and quality of care. While they attached importance to adequate numbers of and well-trained care-givers, they also treasured their decision making and autonomy. There was no hierarchy of importance. Wunderlick and Kohler (2001, p. 30) point out that "efforts to improve one desired outcome (e.g., independence) may compromise another (e.g., avoidance of injury to self or others), and different people may value and balance these and other outcomes differently." If nursing homes that identify with providing resident-centered care find it difficult to practice the duality of quality of care and quality of life, then it is likely that nursing homes with a provider-centered care focus are even less likely to address quality of life issues.

While younger and healthier consumers of long-term care have achieved a greater voice in the provision of their care (Kane & Kane, 2001; Wunderlick & Kohler, 2001), frail older adults are rarely involved in policy making decisions that impact their daily lives. The result can often be elders who withdraw from previously satisfying aspects of life. While many of our study participants retained confidence in their own abilities, a few participants expressed fear that they would make the wrong decisions and looked to staff to make decisions for them. Resident-centered care that focuses on quality of life can assist older adults in nursing home care to retain or even re-find their ability to make choices and decisions that bring satisfaction and quality to their lives. The choice of how involved to be in decision-making needs to remain with the older adult no matter what level of involvement they prefer.

This is an ideal time to address the issue of quality of life for older adults living in nursing homes. While quality of care studies have received the greatest attention and these studies (Harrington, 2002; Report to Congress, 2001), are also raising concerns about staffing and reimbursement, quality of life must be included in the debate about how elders in need of residential care will have their needs met. Numerous inroads have been made regarding care of other populations and in other settings in long-term care. Researchers who study consumer-centered care have found that it is generally practiced in home and community based settings and found less often in skilled nursing facilities (Benjamin & Matthias, 2001; Doty, Kasper, & Litvak, 1996; Litvak, Zukas, & Heumann, 1987; Scala & Mayberry, 1997). These studies can provide a basis for changing the status quo care of frail older adults.

CONCLUSION

While both quality of care and quality of life are important aspects of services to frail elderly living in nursing homes, it is essential to bring attention to the issue of quality of life, which has been overshadowed by quality of care concerns. Both are important to the older adults with whom we spoke. It is essential that they both be emphasized within the conversation about providing nursing home care for older adults.

This study only scratched the surface of quality of life issues for frail elderly living in rural nursing homes. Further studies are needed to identify the continuum of quality of life issues that are important to this population. Finding ways to measure quality of life issues is essential to bring increased emphasis to life satisfaction in a time when outcome measurement dominates policy and resources.

Results of this study underscore the importance of developing policies and procedures that promote decisional control in everyday matters of an older person's life. Results further support the need to advocate for policies that are based on the wants and needs of elders themselves and empower older persons to play a more active role in decision making. NHRA has provided policy helpful to recognize the needs of elders. All of the NHRA directives need to be carried out to support changes in the structure of nursing homes so that they better meet the needs of their residents. Policy that truly supports quality of life requires that all staff be trained to understand what quality of life means. Home is about more than quality of care. As one resident said "I like to come and go as I please. . . . It helps a lot. I feel a whole lot freer."

REFERENCES

Arcus, S.G. (1999). The long-term care ombudsman program: A social work perspective. *Journal of Gerontological Social Work, 31*(1/2), 195-205.

Atchley, R.C., & Barusch, A.S. (2004). *Social forces & aging*. Belmont, CA: Wadsworth/Thomson Learning.

Benjamin, A.E., & Matthias, R.E. (2001). Age, consumer direction, and outcomes of supportive services at home. *The Gerontologist, 41*(5), 632-642.

Butler, R. (1987). Ageism. In G. Maddox (Ed.), *The encyclopedia of aging*. New York: Springer.

Chapin, R., & Cox, E.O. (2001). Changing the paradigm: Strengths-based and empowerment-oriented social work with frail elders. *Journal of Gerontological Social Work, 36*(3/4), 166-179.

Code of Federal Regulations, 42CFR483.15. (2003). *Title 42–Public health–Quality of life*. Washington, DC: U.S. Government Printing Office.

Code of Federal Regulations, 42CFR483.25. (2003). *Title 42–Public health–Quality of care*. Washington, DC: U.S. Government Printing Office.

Cox, C. (1993). *The frail elderly: Problems, needs, and community responses*. Westport, CT: Auburn House.

Cruickshank, M. (2003). *Learning to be old*. Lanham, MD: Rowman & Littlefield Publishers, Inc.

Doty, P., Kasper, J., & Litvak, S. (1996). Consumer-directed models of personal care: Lessons from Medicaid. *Milbank Quarterly, 74*(3), 377-409.

Erikson, E. H., Erikson, J.M., & Kivnick, H.Q. (1986). *Vital involvement in old age*. New York: Norton.

Gatz, M., & Pearson, C.G. (1988). Ageism revised and the provision of psychological services. *American Psychologist, 43*(3), 184-188.

Hagebak, J.E., & Hagebak, B.R. (1983). Meeting the mental health needs of the elderly: Issues and action steps. *Aging, 335-336*, 26-31.

Harrington, C. (2002, June). *Nursing home quality: State agency survey funding and performance*. (Issue Paper). The Kaiser Commission on Medicaid and the Uninsured.

Harvey, G. (2001). The rights of elderly people in a nursing home–A little creativity, a lot of respect, a taste for adventure, and an allergy to bureaucracy. In L.F. Heumann, M.E. McCall, & D.P. Boldy (Eds.), *Empowering frail elderly people* (pp. 155-173). Westport, CT: Praeger Publishers.

Hawes, C. (1997, Fall). Regulation and the politics of long-term care. [Electronic version]. *Generations Journal of the American Society on Aging, 21*(4), 5-12.

Hawes, C., Mor, V., Phillips, C.D., Fries, B.E., Morris, J.N., Steele-Friedlob, E. et al. (1997). The OBRA-87 nursing home regulations and implementation of resident assessment instrument: Effects on process quality. *Journal of the American Geriatrics Society, 45*(8), 997-985.

Hillier, S., & Barrow, G. M. (1999). *Aging, the individual, and society*. Belmont, CA: Wadsworth Publishing Company.

Hillman, J.L., Stricker, G., & Zweig, R.A. (1997). Clinical psychologists' judgments of older adult patients with character pathology implications for practice. *Professional Psychology: Research and Practice, 28*(2), 179-183.

Hinrichsen, G.A., & McMeniman, M. (2002). The impact of geropsychology training. *Professional Psychology: Research and Practice, 33*(3), 337-340.

Hooyman, N. R., & Kiyak, H. A. (2002). *Social gerontology* (6th ed.). Boston: Allyn & Bacon.

Intrieri, R.C., Kelly, J.A., Brown, M.M., & Castilla, C. (1993). Improving medical students' attitudes toward and skills with the elderly. *The Gerontologist, 33*(3), 373-378.

Kane, R. A., Caplan, A. L., Urv-Wong, E. K., Freeman, I. C., Aroskar, M. A., & Finch, M. (1997). Everyday matters in the lives of nursing home residents: Wish for and perception of choice and control. *JAGS, 45*(9), 1086-1093.

Kane, R. L., & Kane, R. A. (2001). What older people want from long-term care and how they can get it. *Health Affairs, 20*(6), 114-127.

Kane, R.L., Williams, C.C., Williams, T.F., & Kane, R.A. (1993). Restraining restraints: Changes in a standard of care. *Annual Review of Public Health, 14*, 545-584.

Kart, C. S., & Kinney, J. M. (2001). *The realities of aging: An introduction to gerontology* (6th ed.). Boston: Allyn & Bacon.

Litvak, S., Zukas, H., & Heumann, J.E. (1987). *Attending to America–Personal assistance for independent living: A survey of attendant service programs in the United States for people of all ages with disabilities.* Berkeley, CA: World Institute on Disability.

Lynott, R.J., & Lynott, P.P. (1996). Tracing the course of theoretical development in the sociology of aging. *The Gerontologist, 36*(6), 749-760.

McInnis-Dittrich, K. (2002). *Social work with elders: A biopsychosocial approach to assessment and intervention* (2nd ed.). Boston: Allyn & Bacon.

Methodist Manor Retirement Community. (2002). *Person-centered care* [Brochure]. Storm Lake, IA: Penniman, T.L.

Mok, B., & Mui, A. (1996). Empowerment in residential care for the elders: The case of an aged home in Hong Kong. *Journal of Gerontological Social Work, 27*(1/2), 23-35.

National Rural Health Association (2001). *Long-term care in rural America.* Retrieved August 1, 2004 from *http://www.nrharural.org/pagefile/issuepapers/ipaper21.html.*

Ouslander, J. G. (1995). The inescapable ethical issues of long-term care. *NH Practitioner, May/June,* 13-17.

Phillips, C., Morris, J.N., Hawes, C., Fries, B.E., Mor, V., Nennstiel, M. et al. (1997). Association of the Resident Assessment Instrument (RAI) with changes in function, cognition and psychosocial status. *Journal of the American Geriatrics Association, 45*(8), 986-993.

Report to Congress: Appropriateness of minimum nurse staffing ratios in nursing homes. (December, 2001) Retrieved August 19, 2004 from Health and Human Services, Centers for Medicare & Medicaid Services Web site: *http://www.cms.hhs.gov/medicaid/reports/rp700hmp.asp?*

Robb, C., Chen, H., & Haley, W.E. (2002, January). Ageism in mental health and health care: A critical review. *Journal of Clinical Geropsychology, 8*(1), 1-12.

Scala, M.A., & Mayberry, P.S. (1997). *Consumer-directed home services: Issues and models.* Oxford, OH: Ohio Long-Term Care Research Project, Miami University.

Teno, J.M., Branco, K.J., Mor, V., Philips, C.D., Hawes, C., & Morris, J. (1997). Changes in advance care planning in nursing homes before and after the patient Self-Determination Act: Report of a 10-state survey. *Journal of the American Geriatric Society, 45*(8), 939-944.

Turner, F.J. (Ed.). (1986). *Social work treatment (3rd ed.).* New York: The Free Press.

Turnham, H. (n.d.). Federal Nursing Home Reform Act from the Omnibus Budget Reconciliation Act of 1987. Retrieved September 14, 2004 from the National Long Term Care Ombudsman Resource Center Web site: *http://www.ltcombudsman.org/ombpublic?PF_251_1348_7568.cfm.*

U.S. Census Bureau (2000). *Group quarters population by sex by age by group quarters.* Retrieved September 14, 2004 from *http//:factfinder.census.gov/servlet/DTTable?_bm=y&geo_id.*

Wunderlich, G.S., & Kohler, P.O. (Eds.). (2001). *Improving the quality of long-term care.* Washington, DC: National Academies Press.

Zhang, X., & Grabowski, D. C. (2004). Nursing home staffing and quality under the Nursing Home Reform Act. *The Gerontologist, 44*(1), 13-23.

Child Abuse Investigation and Treatment for Deaf and Hard of Hearing Children: Ethical Practice and Policy

Emilie Edwards
Jennie Vaughn
Karen Smith Rotabi

SUMMARY. Deaf children are more susceptible than other children to abuse in home and institutional settings. Many helping professionals are unaware of the unique vulnerabilities and needs of the deaf; this lack of awareness limits the effectiveness of their services to that population. Laws and ethical standards mandate that social workers and others use communication methods that deaf clients can understand; however, many human service agencies rely on less than adequate means of communica-

---

Emilie Edwards is a student at the University of North Carolina School of Law.

Jennie Vaughn is affiliated with the UNC School of Social Work, serving as project coordinator for a study about public mental healthcare in North Carolina.

Karen Smith Rotabi, PhD, received her PhD in social work from the UNC School of Social Work in December 2004. She is currently working on a research project at the School of Social Work.

Within Deaf Culture, the words deaf and culture are often capitalized when referring to that collective group. However, to avoid confusion among readers of this article, which largely will be nonmembers of the Deaf Culture, the authors have elected to put these terms in lowercase. This decision was made solely in the interest of clarity and in no way is meant to minimize the significance of the rights and interests of the Deaf.

[Haworth co-indexing entry note]: "Child Abuse Investigation and Treatment for Deaf and Hard of Hearing Children: Ethical Practice and Policy." Edwards, Emilie, Jennie Vaughn, and Karen Smith Rotabi. Co-published simultaneously in *The Social Policy Journal* (The Haworth Press, Inc.) Vol. 4, No. 3/4, 2005, pp. 53-67; and: *Cutting-Edge Social Policy Research* (ed: Richard Hoefer) The Haworth Press, Inc., 2005, pp. 53-67. Single or multiple copies of this article are available for a fee from The Haworth Document Delivery Service [1-800-HAWORTH, 9:00 a.m. - 5:00 p.m. (EST). E-mail address: docdelivery@haworthpress.com].

Available online at http://www.haworthpress.com/web/SPJ

doi:10.1300/J185v04n03_04

tion in child abuse investigations and other procedures. Such ineffective intervention practices fail to protect a vulnerable population of children who literally cannot speak for themselves.

KEYWORDS. Deaf and hard of hearing, child abuse, child abuse investigations, policy, ethical practice, civil rights

Deaf children are substantially more likely than hearing children to suffer physical and/or sexual abuse in home and institutional settings (Berke, n.d.; Bertling, 1994; Elder, 1993b; Embry, unpublished; Mertens, 1996; Sullivan, Scanlan, Brookhouser & Schulte, 1992; Sullivan, Vernon & Scanlan, 1987; Vernon, 1997). Social workers and other helping professionals are as responsible for the welfare of deaf children as they are for that of any other child but in general have little or no knowledge regarding the differing needs of deaf children. This lack of knowledge can lead to less effective intervention practices and, ultimately, failure to protect a vulnerable population of children who literally cannot speak for themselves.

The goal of this article is to establish that methods of communication with deaf clients that have previously been deemed "good enough" are insufficient according to the legal and ethical duties of social workers in child protective service settings. We address the cultural and linguistic backgrounds of deaf Americans and the singular life contexts of the deaf. We address the history of discrimination and disempowerment that perpetuates the inability of deaf clients to advocate for themselves. We outline a variety of legislation granting rights to the deaf. We describe and discuss several communication methods commonly used in practice with deaf clients and explain the legal, ethical, and practical importance of cultural competence and zealous advocacy for this population of children that is particularly vulnerable. We conclude with a discussion of current administrative policy and civil rights issues in child protection services with deaf clients and difficulties in implementation.

INCREASED RISK OF MALTREATMENT FOR DEAF CHILDREN

Abuse in residential schools for the deaf has been well documented and publicized in recent years (Berke, n.d.; Bolstad, 1999; Elder, 1993a, b;

Mertens, 1996; Ombudsman of British Columbia, 1993; Steer, 1998; Sullivan & Knutson, 1989; Sullivan, Vernon, & Scanlan, 1987; Whitlock & Sheehan, 1998; Zezima, 2004). While maltreatment of children in institutional settings is an important issue to explore, it should be noted that a vast majority of deaf children live with their families, and it is in the home that most abuse of deaf children occurs. Some experts estimate that as many as 88 percent of abuse of children with disabilities occurs in the home, most commonly by a family member (Sullivan & Knutson, 1989). Babysitters, clergy, bus drivers, peers, and neighbors also are frequent perpetrators (Sullivan & Knutson, 1989). In this era of deinstitutionalization, deaf children are typically mainstreamed: in 1994, 72 percent of deaf children were educated in typical public school classroom environments and living at home, compared to only 30 percent in 1979 (Allen, 1994). A recent study by Knutson, Johnson, and Sullivan (2004) found that hearing parents of deaf children are significantly more likely to physically abuse these children than are parents of hearing children. Thus, the disturbing trend must be further studied and documented to raise public awareness and promote policy change to protect the deaf.

There are very few formalized studies pertaining to the abuse of deaf children (Bolstad, 1999; Elder, 1993a; Mertens, 1996; Whitlock & Sheehan, 1998; Zezima, 2004). A study of deaf adults–mostly college students–indicated that as many as 50 percent of deaf children are sexually abused before the age of eighteen (Sullivan, Vernon, & Scanlan, 1987; Sullivan & Knutson, 1989). Studies further indicate that 41.6 percent of deaf children are physically abused and that 26 percent of deaf children are neglected (Sullivan & Knutson, 1989). It is important to note, however, that the subjects used in these studies are highly unrepresentative of the deaf population as a whole, as only 4 percent of deaf persons attend college (Allen, 1994). Deaf students tend to display below-average performance in academic settings and are less likely to graduate from high school (Allen, 1994). Children who have experienced abuse and neglect also suffer academically and are less likely to complete high school than children from non-abusive environments (Kinard, 1999; Pecora, Whittaker, Maluccio, & Barth, 2000). The minority of deaf students who do pursue higher education are more likely to have supportive families, adequate financial resources, and adequate access to the educational environment via American Sign Language (ASL) instruction in the classroom, interpreters, cued-speech, etc. (Van Cleve, 1989). It is likely, therefore, that true abuse statistics likely are much higher than those cited above.

REASONS FOR INCREASED RISK OF MALTREATMENT

The reasons for this increased risk of maltreatment have not been extensively studied with the deaf population. Sullivan, Vernon, and Scanlan (1987) theorize that children who have had extensive experience with special education have restricted communication skills. These children also are generally less knowledgeable than hearing children about sexuality and generally have not been trained about personal and sexual boundaries and how to respond to violations of these boundaries (Sullivan, Vernon, & Scanlan, 1987). In addition, deaf children are more conditioned than their hearing counterparts to obey authority figures without questioning them and are more fearful of threats. Finally, even those children who do understand they are being mistreated are less able, because of communication limitations, to raise questions regarding abuse or to report it (Sullivan, Vernon, & Scanlan, 1987).

One particularly problematic issue that arises during child abuse investigations is that deaf culture exerts intense pressure to prevent reports of maltreatment from being shared with hearing service providers, even when a deaf child is being victimized (Ombudsman, 1993; Elder, 1993b; Mertens, 1996; Rubin, 1995). This is particularly true if the abuser is also deaf (Mertens, 1996). This fear stems from anxiety that involving the hearing-based social service agencies may result in a child's removal from the home–and a loss of contact with deaf culture (Elder, 1993b; Mertens, 1996).

Additionally, a strong cultural pressure exists among the deaf to keep their problems out of the public eye (Bertling, 1994; Elder, 1993a, b; Rubin, 1995; Sullivan & Knutson, 1989). Sexual abuse is especially stigmatized, likely a result of the well-documented history of sexual abuse in residential schools for the deaf (Elder, 1993b). In general, the deaf believe that deaf culture is defined by, maintained, and propagated in the residential schools for the deaf and that any threat to the viability of these schools is also a threat to the viability of the culture (Elder, 1993b; Mertens, 1996; Rubin, 1995).

In light of feared the threat to deaf culture, the stigma surrounding disclosure of sexual abuse at deaf residential schools is perhaps understandable. However, this stigma extends to disclosure of such abuse by or against a deaf person in any setting, even those well outside school walls. When *DeafLife* magazine editor Matthew Moore published, in 1994, a story regarding the sexual abuse by neighbors of a 9-year-old deaf child, Benita Vargas, he wrote the following:

> I [am printing this] story . . . to show that deaf children are STILL being neglected and abused, that the system fails to protect them, and that the Deaf community needs to do something about it. . . . There is an old taboo in our community against discussing and publicizing sexual abuse. People know it exists but don't want to talk about it. Our own silence makes it difficult to attack the problem. (Rubin, 1995, p. 9)

Even if stigma were not an issue, most deaf children recognize that hearing adults are unlikely to possess sufficient vocabulary and fluency in sign language to understand a disclosure of abuse (Elder, 1993a). McCay Vernon, a hearing psychologist and prolific researcher in the field of deafness, explains that this is because childhood sign language is so different from the sign language taught in formal ASL courses that many non-deaf ASL speakers are unable to understand the child's cry for help and thus the abuse continues (Elder, 1993a; Sullivan, Vernon, & Scanlan, 1987). Vernon further states his belief that most deaf children do not even attempt to disclose abuse to hearing adults because they know the communication limits of most hearing persons (Elder, 1993b).

DOMINANT PERSPECTIVES REGARDING THE DEAF: THE MEDICAL/PATHOLOGICAL VIEW AND THE CULTURAL VIEW

Understanding deaf culture is as crucial in providing services to deaf clients as is understanding African American or Hispanic culture when providing services to members of these cultural and ethnic groups. Social workers are bound by the National Association of Social Workers (NASW) Code of Ethics (1996) and thus have an ethical duty to achieve understanding and competence with clients from all cultural and ethnic groups (Code of Ethics Section 1.05, 1996). The way in which helping professionals view persons who are deaf and the deaf community as a whole can have a huge impact on their ability to provide real help to this population of clients. It was in only the 1970s that sociologists and linguists in the United States began to recognize the existence of a distinct deaf culture (Lane, 1999), and understanding among the hearing remains incomplete.

The *medical/pathological view* (Humphrey & Alcorn, 1994) is defined as "an attitude based on pathological thinking which results in a negative stigma toward anyone who does not hear; like racism or sexism, audism judges, labels, and limits individuals on the basis of whether a person hears and speaks" (1994, p. 85). This view stems from a belief often found in in-group/out-group dynamics (Jansson, 2003), that the dominant culture is "normal," "standard," and/or "right" and that the minority culture is "deviant," "inadequate," and/or "wrong" (Lane, 1999).

More accepting and inclusive is the *cultural view* in which the deaf community is seen as a group of persons "who share a common means of communication (sign language) that provides the basis for group cohesion and identity, . . . who share a common language (ASL) and a common culture, . . . [and] whose primary means of relating to the world is visual and who share a language that is visually received and gesturally produced" (Sign Media Inc., n.d.).

The cultural view is the more appropriate perspective by which social workers should view the deaf community as it is more consistent with the way members of this community typically view themselves. This cultural view is a strengths-based perspective (Saleeby, 1997); as such, it could be asserted that the deaf client's culture of origin has the potential to serve as a support system. Thus, deaf clients may be able to derive greater stability and gain resilience through their connection to deaf culture. Unfortunately, this inclusive nature of deaf culture may be a double-edged sword; those who may need to escape oppression or abuse perpetuated by those within the culture may quickly come to view the community's cozy insularity as a stifling trap. These and other dynamics must be considered when conducting investigations regarding abuse of children who are deaf (Bertling, 1994).

DIFFERING LIFE EXPERIENCES, EDUCATIONAL CONTEXTS, AND CULTURAL PERSPECTIVES OF PERSONS WHO ARE DEAF

Being deaf is different from being a member of another cultural or ethnic minority in that unless a deaf person lives at a residential school for the deaf, s/he likely has access to few, if any, persons who are fluent in their language, sign language. Conversely, members of most other minority groups generally have access to family and/or friends with whom they can communicate in their native language. Deafness is different from other conditions in that it separates the deaf person from communication in a unique way. Helen Keller once stated: "Blindness cuts people off from *things,* while deafness cuts people off from other *people.* The inability to communicate may result in depression or psychosis" (Rubin, 1995, p. 10; italics added by authors).

The deaf community in the United States has its own set of values and mores. Most importantly, deaf culture does not view deafness as a disability (Bertling, 1994; Franklin, 2004; Humphrey & Alcorn, 1994; Lane, 1999; Padden & Humphries, 1988; Saks, 1989). Some deaf persons, especially those who identify as "Strong Deaf," view with disdain deaf persons who prefer communication methods other than ASL (i.e., speech/lip reading, cued speech, and non-ASL forms of sign language that attempt to code English onto the hands), who use hearing aids, or who have cochlear implants (Franklin, 2004; Lane, 1999; Padden & Humphries, 1988). Deaf culture takes pride in deafness and devalues those who attempt to function as if they were hearing (Franklin, 2004; Humphrey & Alcorn, 1994; Lane, 1999; Padden & Humphries, 1988).

The life experiences of deaf clients are tremendously different than those of hearing clients. Some of these differences are experiential (Franklin, 2004; Padden & Humphries, 1988; Saks, 1989), educational (Berke, n.d.; Lane, 1999), and linguistic (Elder, 1993a; Saks, 1989), in addition to the aforementioned cultural differences. Of the five senses, humans gain more information about how to behave, how to communicate, and how to respond to stimuli from hearing and seeing (Bandura, 1986). Hearing children gain a great deal of information through casual aural stimuli, while deaf children miss out on these learning opportunities. For example, most children begin to learn about sex and sexuality–including the difference between appropriate and inappropriate touch–by talking with their peers (Haffner, 2004). However, deaf children in typical public school environments do not have access to such discussions.

Another major source of information acquisition for hearing people is reading. Most people erroneously assume that because deaf people have unimpaired vision they are able to gain information through reading and to convey information through writing (Myers & Thyer, 1997). Education curricula are typically designed with the assumption that the student already possesses a firm verbal grasp of at least one language. In the U.S., children entering formal educational settings are expected to be able to speak and understand spoken English. (Children not fluent in English are placed in English as a Second Language (ESL) classes, which are heavily oral (Huddelson, Italiano, & Rounds, 1993).

For most hearing children, language skills are obtained effortlessly. From infancy, their environment is saturated with the spoken word as they are constantly exposed to the voices of their parents, siblings, and other care providers, as well as sounds from television, radio, and other media. These aural stimuli are not available to deaf children. Ninety percent of deaf children are born to hearing parents (Gaulladet Research Institute, 2003). Since most hearing people do not use any type of sign language, there is a risk that deaf children will receive little or no language stimuli during their early years. Additionally, many deaf children are not identified as deaf until late infancy and thus have missed out on prophylactic measures to prevent language delays (Simeonsson, 2003).

Some states have begun to incorporate hearing tests into neonatal health exams. While this policy is extremely helpful in preventing language delays, it is not consistently applied. Many deaf children who enter child protection investigations have not had these exams and are thus still likely to have experienced or be experiencing difficulty with communication of any type. When these children are exposed to sign language, they acquire it easily (Saks, 1989). However, when oral education is emphasized over sign language acquisition, the comprehension of spoken English is substantially delayed (Lane, 1999).

This barrier to English acquisition creates a further barrier to the acquisition of reading skills, which in turn greatly hinders future academic success. Instruction in hearing-integrated classrooms, which relies largely on oral skills and phonics, does not provide most deaf children a strong enough foundation in English to enable them to learn to read (Lane, 1999). The average reading level of a deaf high school graduate in the United States is between the third and fourth grade (Lane, 1999). This lower literacy level does not indicate an intellectual deficit; it indicates only that pedagogical methods for deaf children are highly inferior.

Perhaps one reason for this disparity is the vast linguistic differences in the communications used by the hearing and the deaf. Most people believe that American Sign Language (ASL) is manually coded English, that there is a corresponding sign for each English word, and that concepts will translate directly. This is not true. ASL is a unique system of communication with its own grammar, syntax, and structure (Saks, 1989) which differs significantly from English. It is a completely visual language with its own metaphors and language-based humor. Despite its name, ASL resembles English *less* than do Spanish, French, or German. Yet while no social worker or other helping professional would consider conducting a maltreatment investigation with a Spanish-speaking client without a translator, service providers frequently conduct child protection investigations with ASL users relying on English only, and without any concrete verification that the ASL user possesses sufficient English skills to fully participate in communication.

A frequently used expression in ASL is "Train go sorry"; the English translation is "Sorry, you missed it." The deaf experience is so full of these "train go sorry" incidents that this phrase was used as the title of a popular book about the deaf experience (Cohen, 1994). People who are deaf become used to living in a world of partial information and understanding, a world in which nodding, smiling, and going along with half-understood cues is the easiest course of action. While this may be permissible in some situations, it must not be allowed with the helping professions.

The NASW Code of Ethics (1996) expressly prohibits social workers from relying on the deaf client to accept the "train go sorry" experience in social work settings because of the profession's commitment to self-determination and duty to aid in a competent manner. According to Section 1.03, social workers must use "clear and understandable language [in communication with] clients" and that clients who are unable to fully comprehend and express themselves in the language used by the social worker must be provided with a "qualified interpreter" (NASW, 1996). These ethical requirements proscribe that social workers must honor the client's perspective by interviewing that client using whatever means are most comfortable for the client and going to all necessary lengths to ensure that the client understands what is happening, even when doing so may cause inconvenience or additional expense.

ANTI-DISCRIMINATION STATUTES AND THE ETHICAL VALUES OF INCLUSION AND CULTURAL COMPETENCE

Child protection laws and abuse investigation procedures vary widely from state to state and depending on the perceived risk and severity of the alleged maltreatment. Regardless of jurisdiction, however, social workers are ethically bound by duty to consistently deliver the most competent and comprehensive service possible to every client. Section 4.02 of the NASW Code of Ethics states that "[s]ocial workers should not practice, condone, facilitate, or collaborate with any form of discrimination on the basis of . . . mental or physical disability" (1996). To settle for less than an optimum degree of communication with clients is unethical because to do so is to facilitate and collaborate with discriminatory practices.

A number of legal statutes and court decisions establish the right to equal access to meaningful communication for deaf clients. Among the legal statutes are Executive Order 13166 signed by President Bill Clinton in 1996, Titles II and III of the Americans with Disabilities Act (ADA) ratified in 1990, Public Law 504 of 1978, Titles I, III, and V of the Rehabilitation Act of 1973, and Title VI of the Civil Rights Act of 1964. The scope of this paper does not allow for a detailed treatment of these statutes and orders, but their summative order is that service providers must not, in any avoidable way, allow disability or limited English proficiency to hinder their work with deaf clients. Communication must be completely accessible to deaf participants in social service settings.

Ethical practice requires that social workers become civil rights advocates when working with disempowered populations such as the deaf (NASW, Section 2.03,1996). The deaf have little experience advocating for themselves for a variety of reasons. The first has to do with access to communication with the agents of the courts.

The Americans with Disabilities Act (ADA) guarantees deaf people the right to interpreters in court. Persons who are deaf also have the right to a court-appointed attorney when charged with a crime. However, if a deaf person wishes to hire a private attorney, no such attorney is required to accept his or her case. Interpreters are frequently required to facilitate client-attorney communication during trial preparation, as most deaf people do not have sufficient English skills to explain their needs to hearing attorneys. Paying for these costly interpreter services substantially decreases the financial incentive for attorneys to take on these cases of the deaf and therefore decreases the probability that attorneys will take on these cases. Also, while there is a legal advocacy center for the deaf in the United States (the National Association of the Deaf Law Center in Maryland) this single agency has limited funding and personnel. Thus, most complaints involving civil rights violations against the deaf have never reached a courtroom. This pattern of failure to litigate breaches of civil rights results in a substantial weakening of anti-discrimination laws.

COMMUNICATION METHODS AND ACCOMMODATIONS AS SUGGESTED BY THE ADA

Persons who are deaf receive all communication visually, generally by observing the speaker's lips, via written communication or pictures, or with sign language. Sign language is by far the easiest method of communication for deaf persons to perceive fully (Saks, 1989). The use of speech and lip-reading is the least effective (Humphreys & Alcorn, 1994). Unfortunately, the lip-reading skills of most deaf children, especially younger ones, are not yet fully developed, and reading and writing are out of the question.

The ADA requires that reasonable accommodations be made for persons with disabilities (DiNitto, 2003) and lists several possible methods of communicating with deaf clients. One of the methods specified is lip-reading for those deaf clients who are skilled in that area. While it is widely assumed that deaf persons are highly adept at lip-reading, a deaf person, even with extensive training, can read lips only as well as the average hearing person (Lane, 1999). Such incomplete communication is a serious liability to child abuse investigations considering the ethical and practical importance of complete understanding for all persons involved.

It is interesting to note that only 30 percent of English is visible on the lips (Humphrey & Alcorn, 1994; Lane, 1999; Padden & Humphries, 1988; Saks, 1989). Perception is compromised even further by poor lighting, fatigue, and emotional distress. Considering the degree of developmental delay that occurs in abused and neglected children and their relative inexperience with lip-reading, the inadequacy of this method of communication becomes apparent.

Another option recommended by the ADA for communication with deaf persons is writing notes. Unfortunately, the literacy skills of most deaf persons fall far below the average because most deaf children are taught to read using methods that rely on the ability to hear. Thus, corresponding via the written word is also a poor choice of communication for most deaf adults and is rarely even an option for deaf children, most of whom have only rudimentary writing skills at best (Kinard, 1999; Pecora et al., 2000). Relying on finger spelling is also unacceptable.

The final choice suggested by the ADA for communicating with deaf clients is the use of a "qualified interpreter," defined as "someone who can interpret effectively, accurately, and impartially both receptively and expressively using any specialized vocabulary" (ADA, 1990). Especially key is complete impartiality, which means that the interpreter should have no vested interest in the outcome of the case. In a child protective services setting, it is unacceptable to allow schoolteachers, educational interpreters, church members, friends, and family members of anyone involved in the investigation to serve as an interpreter, as they may embellish or disregard statements that they do not want to hear or believe. Potential bias by a partial interpreter can invalidate the entire contents of an interview.

Accurately interpreting between the hearing and the deaf requires that the interpreter have more than a clear grasp of ASL grammar and syntax and an extensive vocabulary. The interpreter must also be attuned to the linguistic functioning of deaf clients and must alter their own tone of communication to match. The interpreter's tone matching skill is similar to the social worker's skill at selecting different terminology and breaking down concepts in different ways for different clients. Like others involved in child protection investigations, they must not confuse children with large words or complex sentences nor condescend to educated adults by speaking in overly simplistic terms. Additionally, they must understand the adult who uses scientifically correct terms for parts of the anatomy as easily as they understand the child who uses slang or baby terms. Most of this vocabulary is not taught in standard ASL classes; it is generally covered only in specialized certification programs.

Familiarity with specialized vocabulary is a particularly difficult standard to achieve when one considers the implications of tone. There are no specific signs for many of the terms used in maltreatment investigations. Instead, many ASL users will resort to finger-spelling the English word. While this may work for some deaf adults (though it is far from ideal), it is unacceptable as a means of communicating with deaf children. Instead, the interpreter must be sufficiently familiar with the social service setting that they can break the English vocabulary into its conceptual components, then convey them in a tone appropriate for the client. The level of skill in the English language, ASL, and tone-modulation that is required to effectively and accurately convey the specialized concepts involved in child protection investigations should be trusted only to the highest caliber of interpreters.

CONCLUSION

Social workers and other helping professionals, such as child protection case managers, are inherently committed to advocacy and appropriate treatment for children and families but are constrained by their reality of heavy workloads and insufficient funding (Kinard, 1999; Pecora et al., 2000). In this current environment of resource-scarcity, locating and paying for qualified interpreters places a significant burden on most child protection agencies. This reality creates additional risks for deaf clients and puts some of our society's most vulnerable children at risk for re-traumatization. Despite repeated documentation of violations of the rights of the deaf, the provision of competent human services through the use of qualified interpreters remains an unfunded mandate. This problem is further complicated by the fact that there is no national system to track child protection cases involving the deaf. For example, the state of North Carolina does not gather data regarding hearing status of children involved in abuse investigations (personal communication, Joanne Lamm, North Carolina Director of Child Protective Services, November, 2003). As a result, it is impossible to quantify the number of deaf children and families who enter the child protection system so that their needs can be recognized and budgeted for.

A simple retooling of health and child protection policy could effect significant improvements for deaf persons and their families. A national mandate for neonatal hearing tests would result in early intervention for deaf children and education for their parents regarding nonverbal forms of communication. Such a mandate would also facilitate the recording of this important piece of demographic data so that deaf children and their families can be counted and thus better served. Social work schools should incorporate cultural competence instruction regarding the deaf, and licensing boards should require continuing education regarding deaf issues for all helping professionals, especially those in child protection agencies. Finally, policymakers should mandate and enforce requirements that professional, qualified ASL interpreters be on hand for all child protective services interviews involving deaf children and/or families. These interpreters can be hired through the National Association for the Deaf (NAD) or the Registry of Interpreters for the Deaf (RID).

Child protection laws and the NASW Code of Ethics require that competent social workers more effectively intervene on behalf of deaf children and their families and develop better practices for follow-up treatment. Failure to do so amounts to nothing less than unlawful discrimination. Deaf people deserve to receive the same human and social services that are provided to the hearing; our nation's civil rights laws require it. The needs of deaf Americans will not change but our response to them must.

REFERENCES

Allen, T. E. (1994). Who are the deaf and hard-of-hearing students leaving high school and entering postsecondary education? Retrieved July 23, 2004, from the Gallaudet University Graduate Research Institute website, *http://gri.gallaudet.edu/AnnualSurvey/whodeaf.html.*

Bandura, A. (1986). *Social foundations of thought and action: A social cognitive theory.* Englewood Cliffs, NJ: Prentice-Hall.

Berke, J. (n.d.). Sexual abuse of deaf students in schools. Retrieved September 23, 2004, from *http://deafness.about.com/cs/educationgeneral/a/sexabuse.htm.*

Bertling, T. (1994). *A child sacrificed to deaf culture.* Wilsonville, OR: Kodak Media Group.

Bolstad, E. (1999, June 17). Teacher is charged with abuse: A Greensboro teacher at the N.C. School for the Deaf is charged with sexually abusing a female student in 1998. *Greensboro (N.C.) News & Record.* B1.

Cohen, L. H. (1994). *Train go sorry: Inside a deaf world.* New York: Vintage Books.

DiNitto, D. (2003). *Social welfare: Politics and public policy* (5th ed.). Boston: Pearson Education.

Elder, M. (1993a). Abused because of deafness? *Moving Forward* 2(5). Retrieved September 23, 2004, from *http://movingforward.org/v2n5-coverside.html.*

Elder, M. (1993b). Deaf survivors of sexual abuse: A look at the issues. *Moving Forward* 2(5). Retrieved September 23, 2004, from *http://movingforward.org/v2n5-coverside.html.*

Embry, R. A. (2000). *An examination of risk factors for the maltreatment of deaf children.* Unpublished doctoral dissertation, University of California, Berkeley.

Franklin, H. (2004). Straddling the fence. Retrieved September 23, 2004, from the National Association of the Deaf website, *http://www.nad.org.*

Gallaudet Research Institute. (2003). Regional and National Summary Report of Data from the 2002-2003 Annual Survey of Deaf and Hard of Hearing Children and Youth. Washington, DC: Graduate Research Institute, Gallaudet University. Retrieved September 20, 2004, from the Gallaudet University Graduate Research Institute website, *http://gri.gallaudet.edu/Demographics/2003_National_Summary.pdf.*

Haffner, D. W. (2004). *From diapers to dating: A parent's guide to raising sexually healthy children–From infancy to middle school* (2nd ed.). New York: Newmarket.

Huddelson, S., Italiano, G., & Rounds, P. (Eds.). (1993). *English as a Second Language curriculum resource handbook: A practical guide for K-12 ESL programs.* Millwood, NY: Kraus International.

Humphrey, J. H., & Alcorn, B. J. (1994). *So you want to be an interpreter: An introduction to sign language interpreting.* Amarillo, TX: Sign Enhancers.

Jansson, B. S. (2003). *Becoming an effective policy advocate: From policy practice to social justice* (4th ed.). Pacific Grove, CA: Brooks/Cole.

Kinard, E. M. (1999). Psychosocial resources and academic performance in abused children. *Children and Youth Service Review, 21*(5), 351-376.

Knutson, J. F., Johnson, C. R., & Sullivan, P. M. (2004). Disciplinary choices of mothers of deaf children and mothers of normally hearing children. *Child Abuse & Neglect, 28*(9), 925-937.

Lane, H. (1999). *The mask of benevolence: Disabling the deaf community*. New York: DawnSign Press.

Mertens, D. (1996). Breaking the silence about sexual abuse of deaf youth. *American Annals of the Deaf 141*(5): 352-358.

Myers, L., & Thyer, B. (1997). Social work practice with deaf clients: Issues in culturally competent assessment. *Social Work in Health Care 26*(1): 61-76.

National Association of Social Workers. (1996). *NASW Code of Ethics*. Washington, DC: NASW Press.

Ombudsman of British Columbia. (1993, November). Abuse of deaf students at Jericho Hill School. Ombudsman of British Columbia Public Report 32. Retrieved September 23, 2004, from *http://www.ombud.gov.bc.ca/reports/Public_Reports/PR32_Jericho_Hill_School.html*

Padden, C., & Humphries, T. (1988). *Deaf in America: Voices from a culture*. Cambridge: Harvard University Press.

Pecora, P. J., Whittaker, J. K., Maluccio, A. N., & Barth, R. P. (2000). *The child welfare challenge* (2nd ed.). New York: Aldine De Gruyter.

Rubin, P. (1995). The ordeal of Benita Venegas. *DeafLife*, *7*(12), 9-22.

Saks, O. (1989). *Seeing voices: A journey into the world of the deaf*. Berkeley: University of California Press.

Saleeby, D. (1997). *The strengths perspective in social work practice* (2nd ed.). White Plains, NY: Longman.

Sign Media, Inc. (n.d.). American deaf culture. Retrieved on September 20, 2004, from the Sign Media, Inc. [producer of information regarding deaf culture] website, *http://www.signmedia.com/info/adc.htm*.

Simeonsson, R. J. (2003). Classification of communication disabilities in children: Contribution of the International Classification on Functioning, Disability, and Health. *International Journal of Audiology*, *42*(5, Supplement1): S2-S8.

Steer, M. (1998). Abuse of children who are deaf or hard of hearing. *Canadian Association of Educators of the Deaf and Hard of Hearing [CAEDHH] Journal/La Revue ACESM 24*(2/3): 114-117.

Sullivan, P. M., & Knutson, J. F. (1989). Maltreatment and behavioral characteristics of youth who are deaf and hard-of-hearing. *Sexuality and Disability 16*(4): 295-317.

Sullivan, P. M., Scanlan, J. M., Brookhouser, P. E., & Schulte, L. E. (1992). The effects of psychotherapy on behavior problems of sexually abused deaf children. *Child Abuse & Neglect*, *16*(2), 297-307.

Sullivan, P. M., Vernon, M., & Scanlan, J. M. (1987). Sexual abuse of deaf youth. *American Annals of the Deaf*, *132*(4): 256-262.

Van Cleve, J. V. (1989). *A place of their own: Creating the deaf community in America*. Washington, DC: Gaulladet University Press.

Whitlock, C., & Sheehan, R. (1998, June 7). Deaf students' sex-abuse reports handled poorly. *The (Raleigh, N.C.) News & Observer*. A1.

Zezima, K. (2004, May 12). Nine students at school for deaf say they were abused by nuns. *New York Times*. A20.

Connecting Policy to Practice: Analyzing the Variables of the Section 8 Housing Program Policy Process

Barbra A. Teater
David C. Kondrat

SUMMARY. Eight variables affect the policy process of the Section 8 housing program. An analysis of the eight variables allows for conceptualization of the factors influencing the shape and direction that Section 8 policy has taken through the course of history. Examining the variables of the Section 8 housing program can lead to an understanding of the program as a whole, the impact of the policy process on the recipients of the program, and the impact on social work practice. In addition, an understanding of these eight variables provides a useful heuristic for social workers engaged in policy changing activities. *[Article copies available for a fee from The Haworth Document Delivery Service: 1-800-HAWORTH. E-mail address: <docdelivery@haworthpress.com> Website: <http://www.HaworthPress.com> © 2005 by The Haworth Press, Inc. All rights reserved.]*

KEYWORDS. Housing policy, Section 8, social work practice, policy analysis

---

Barbra A. Teater and David C. Kondrat are affiliated with The Ohio State University, College of Social Work, 1947 College Road, 200N Still Hall, Columbus, OH 43210.

[Haworth co-indexing entry note]: "Connecting Policy to Practice: Analyzing the Variables of the Section 8 Housing Program Policy Process." Teater, Barbra, A., and David C. Kondrat. Co-published simultaneously in *The Social Policy Journal* (The Haworth Press, Inc.) Vol. 4, No. 3/4, 2005, pp. 69-92; and: *Cutting-Edge Social Policy Research* (ed: Richard Hoefer) The Haworth Press, Inc., 2005, pp. 69-92. Single or multiple copies of this article are available for a fee from The Haworth Document Delivery Service [1-800-HAWORTH, 9:00 a.m. - 5:00 p.m. (EST). E-mail address: docdelivery@haworthpress.com].

Available online at http://www.haworthpress.com/web/SPJ

doi:10.1300/J185v04n03_05

Social policies are intimately tied to social work practice. As Blau and Abramovitz (2004) make clear, the programs that are available to clients, the services that clients receive, and the benefits that clients are eligible for, are related to social policies. Additionally, social work practice, such as linkage between client and services or resources, is often determined by the availability and accessibility of social programs. Therefore, an understanding of the connection between social policy and social work practice is critical as the effectiveness of social work practice is contingent on the provisions outlined in social polices.

The Section 8 housing program is dictated by a social policy that affects many low-income households in the United States as well as impacts social work practice. The Section 8 housing program is the largest social policy for housing in the United States and serves 1.8 million households (Department of Housing and Urban Development [HUD], 2004). Housing is a vital resource and basic need for individuals and families. Yet, finding affordable housing is difficult for many in the United States. The median sales price for a single-family dwelling unit is $170,000, and the median gross rent with utilities is $691 a month (Joint Center for Housing Studies [JCHS], 2004). Housing is often the largest expense for a household with nearly one-third of Americans spending 30% of their income on housing and 13% spending more than 50% of their income (JCHS, 2004). Additionally, 2.5-3.5 million people are estimated to be homeless in a given year, and 850,000 people are estimated to be homeless on any given night (JCHS, 2004). Based on the difficulties facing low-income households in attaining and maintaining affordable housing, an analysis of the Section 8 housing program is necessary to determine how the largest federal housing program is meeting the needs of low-income households, how the program impacts social work practice, as well as where and by what means social workers can/should intervene to impact future housing policy.

This paper describes the variables of the Section 8 policy process that contribute to an understanding of the shape and content of the Section 8 housing program. Understanding the variables that contribute to Section 8 housing policy and program implementation allow for social work practitioners to impact future Section 8 housing policy and program implementation by helping them conceptualize where and how to intervene. The eight variables identified as contributing to the shape and content of the Section 8 policy process and program will be described. In addition, a link will be made between potential avenues that social work practitioners can use to make future policy and program changes.

HISTORY OF SUBSIDIZED TENANT-BASED HOUSING

The federal government first became involved in the housing of American people through the establishment of the Federal Housing Administration (FHA) in 1934. The prominent American dream of homeownership coupled with the devastating economic effects of the Great Depression prompted the federal government to create the FHA. The FHA insures home mortgage loans which makes homeownership more accessible to individuals and families. For those who could not qualify for a loan, the Housing Act of 1937 created public housing to act as a temporary housing system for low-income families until home- ownership could become attainable. In addition to temporarily housing low-income individuals and families, public housing was enacted to stimulate the economy through housing construction, employment creation, and clearance of slum and blighted areas (Bartelt, 1993; Gotham & Wright, 2000). Public housing remained the central federal low-income housing program for nearly forty years.

The Great Society and War on Poverty initiatives, developed by President Kennedy, and later President Johnson, led to a proposal of subsidized tenant-based housing in the 1960s (Congressional Quarterly [CQ], 1961, 1964, 1965). The Great Society focused on three specific areas in the United States: (a) cities; (b) countryside; and (c) classrooms (CQ, 1964). Urban Renewal signified the transformation of slum and blighted inner-cities into a "Great Society." To tackle the relocation of families affected by urban renewal, the promotion of subsidized tenant-based housing was proposed to ensure relocated families had necessary housing options. The use of the private market widened the housing opportunities of families unexpectedly relocating. A very controversial program, subsidized tenant-based housing was viewed as a "wide-open, socialistic subsidy formula" by several Republicans and conservative Democrats (CQ, 1965, p. 371). The ability of low-income families to rent housing in the private market and potentially position themselves in close proximity to higher-income families, left Republicans and conservative Democrats quite uneasy, as they did not want to interfere with existing social patterns within neighborhoods (CQ, 1965). Despite the opposition from political groups, subsidized tenant-based housing was at last established on August 22, 1974 through the Housing and Community Development Act of 1974 (PL 93-383).

SECTION 8 HOUSING

Section 8 housing is the prominent federal housing program serving 1.8 million low-income households nationwide (HUD, 2004). Section 8 housing vouchers enable recipients to rent housing in the private market versus renting from the federal government. Recipients of Section 8 housing are responsible for paying no more than 30% of their income towards rent, with the federal government providing the remaining balance up to an approved rental amount, referred to as Fair Market Rent (FMR), established for a given geographical area. The FMR, established by the Department of Housing and Urban Development (HUD), includes the cost of utilities (except telephone), and varies by unit size (number of bedrooms). Program eligibility is based on household income with at least 75% of families admitted to the voucher program during the local Public Housing Authority (PHA) fiscal year consisting of extremely low-income families (income not exceeding 30% of the median income for the established geographical area). Current distribution of Section 8 recipients by income includes 68% extremely low income, 17% very low income (50% of the median), and 2% low income (80% of the median) (HUD, 2004).

Policy Goals for Section 8 Housing

The Housing and Community Development Act of 1974 established the Section 8 housing program "for the purpose of aiding lower-income families in obtaining a decent place to live and of promoting economically mixed housing . . ." (42 USC 1435(f) Sec. 8 (a). In addition to promoting mixed-income neighborhoods, Section 8 housing provides recipients with housing mobility and housing choice (U.S. House, 2003). Recipients are able to select housing of their choice in neighborhoods of their choice with the freedom to move to different neighborhoods, pending availability of housing and receiving landlords.

THE SECTION 8 HOUSING PROGRAM POLICY MODEL

The Section 8 housing program policy model is constructed from a historical review of housing policies through the Catalogue of Federal Domestic Assistance (CFDA) and the Congressional Quarterly Almanacs (1946-2002). The eight variables that construct a continual policy process for the Section 8 housing program were derived from identification of significant housing legislation pertinent to subsidized tenant-based housing, review of congressional hearings around identified significant housing legislation, and a thorough review of the Code of Federal Regulations (CFR) and an urban Midwestern PHA's administrative plan in regard to implementation.

The policy process can be described as a circular process (see Figure 1) as the eight variables have and continue to illustrate the shape and content of the Section 8 housing program, which explain the incremental policy changes from 1974 through 2003. An intervention into one (or more) of the eight variables have impacted and continues to impact the shape and content of the program, yet the remaining seven variables are vital to the program's continual existence because the presence of all eight variables are critical in determining the shape and content of the program.

Economic and Social Factors

Two main objectives that consistently contribute to the creation of housing policy include the encouragement of homeownership, and the use of housing to stimulate the economy and alleviate social ills (Mitchell, 1985). In the 1930s, the effects of the Great Depression spurred the federal government to uphold these objectives and use housing to: (a) stimulate construction to increase employment; (b) provide and maintain a

FIGURE 1. Section 8 Housing Program as Circular Policy Process

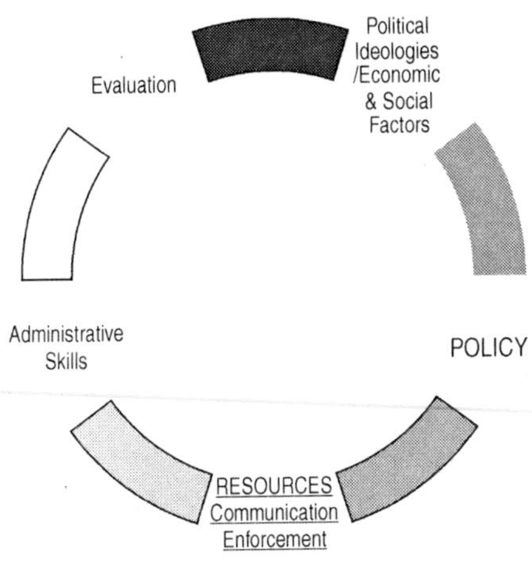

sufficient supply of mortgage credit; and (c) increase the supply of "better" housing to meet the needs of the American people (U.S. Senate, 1974). In times of economic recessions, the federal government has intervened to stimulate the housing market, thereby creating a chain-effect of stimulation to other critical areas of the economy, such as construction, employment, and demand of consumer goods (U.S. House, 1974). The federal government additionally became involved in housing through the (a) acknowledgement of slums and blighted areas in inner cities with goals of slum-clearance and urban renewal; (b) social ills attributed to concentrations of poverty; and (c) housing recessions.

The creation of housing policy, both past and present, consist of the presence of at least one of the above-mentioned economic and/or social factors. For example, the Housing Act of 1937 created public housing with additional goals of clearing the slums that plagued the inner-cities, increasing employment through the building of public housing facilities, increasing the demand of construction materials and consumer goods, and thus, moving the economy out of the recession (Bartelt, 1993; Gotham & Wright, 2000; U.S. House, 1974). Additionally, the 1960s addressed the goal of urban renewal to meet three basic national objectives: (a) to renew cities and assure the sound growth of rapidly expanding metropolitan areas; (b) to provide decent housing for all people; and (c) to encourage a prosperous and efficient construction industry as an essential component of general economic prosperity and growth (CQ, 1961). In the mid-1970s, the longest and most severe housing recession was in existence since World War II (CQ, 1974). One means to combat the housing recession was to enable and encourage households to rent housing in the private market. The federal government turned to subsidized tenant-based housing programs to stimulate the housing industry and reverse the effects of the housing recession.

In combination with the severe housing recession, subsidized tenant-based housing was initiated in the 1970s to promote mixed-income neighborhoods and decrease the social ills attributed to public housing facilities and poverty concentrated neighborhoods. Such social ills can include high crime rates, drug usage, unemployment (Kleit, 2001; Hartung & Henig, 1997) teenage pregnancy, and lack of adequate education (Crane, 1991). Thus, the presence and acknowledgment of economic and social factors, such as economic and housing recessions, and concentrations of poverty and social ills has contributed to the federal government's involvement in housing and the creation and continued promotion of subsidized tenant-based housing.

Political Ideologies

Political ideology is crucial in determining the development of policy and policy programs, as the acting political system produces policies and policy programs in congruence with the prevailing paradigm. Lindblom (1968) defines ideology as an "interlocked set of important generalizations about social organization, or . . . a more formal and highly organized set of such beliefs, like the Marxist-Leninist principles" (p. 23). Karger and Stoesz (2002) define ideology as a "set of assumptions about how the world works: what has value, what is worth living and dying for, what is good and true, and what is right" (p. 6). Political ideologies are not static, but instead tend to change and evolve based on the perceptions and experiences of the decision-makers within the political system (Edelman, 1971). Decision-makers make decisions based on what they believe to be true and best; whether to meet their personal agendas, or to meet the agendas of individuals or groups. Decision-makers believe their decision to be rational as the decision comes about through their experiences and perceptions created through the influence of their environment and culture (Edelman, 1971).

Political ideology plays a critical role in the creation of housing policy and particularly subsidized tenant-based housing policy, as two central questions are asked: (a) Should the federal government become involved in the housing of the American people?; and (b) How should the federal government become involved in the housing of the American people? The answers to these two questions reflect two continuums: (a) the responsibility of the state versus personal responsibility; and (b) an income problem versus a supply problem. A two-by-two table depicts the relationship between these two continuums with each quadrant yielding a particular type, or particular era of housing policy.

An income problem to housing policy identifies that low-income individuals and families do not have a sufficient amount of income to purchase adequate housing. Often, if safe and decent housing is obtained, the low-income individual or family foregoes other living necessities in order to stabilize the housing; many times paying more than 25 percent of their income towards rent (U.S. Senate, 1974). The potential to purchase decent and safe housing increases as the household's income increases. A supply problem to housing acknowledges and accepts that the housing supply is not adequate to provide decent and safe housing for all the nation's citizens (U.S. Senate, 1974). An inadequate supply of housing demonstrates a supply problem, thus proposing solutions that focus on increasing the supply of housing and avoiding considering the necessary income to afford the housing. Instead of treating the root cause of the problem, the inability to pay for housing, the symptom is treated by supplying housing (CQ, 1973).

Although Figure 2 is depicted by a two-by-two table, the type of responsibility and type of problem tend to operate as a continuum. Rarely, throughout the history of housing policy, do the political ideologies that contribute to the type of housing policy and programs neatly fit into one of the four quadrants. The policies and programs move about each quadrant based on how much personal or state responsibility dominates in the ideology of the particular era or political administration combined with the ideological view of the housing problem as either supply or income. Placed within each quadrant in Figure 2 is a particular era in housing policy in which prevailing political ideologies contributed to particular types of housing policy and programs.

Quadrant 2 of Figure 2 depicts the era of state responsibility and a supply problem. Until the Great Depression of the 1930s, the federal government was not involved in the housing of the American people because attainment of housing was viewed as a personal responsibility. During the Great Depression, policymakers realized that involvement in housing would prove beneficial by pushing the economy out of the Depression. Families who under "normal" economic times could potentially afford and/or attain housing could no longer achieve the higher

FIGURE 2. Political Ideology of Housing Policy Eras on Continuums of Responsibility and Source of Problem

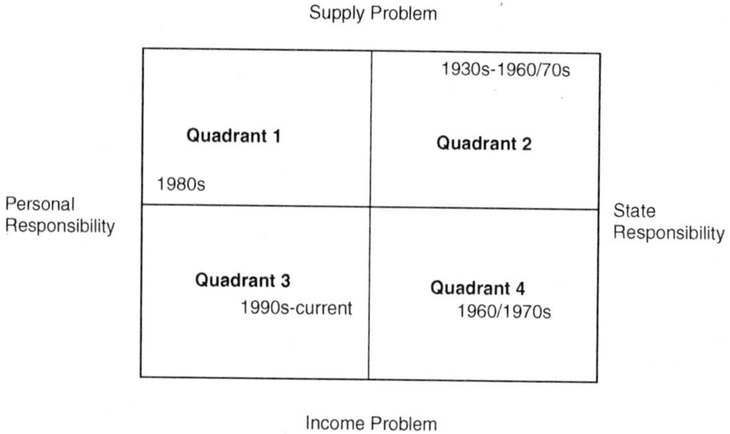

status that homeownership provided. Thus, the federal government assumed responsibility and initiated several housing programs to assist families with their housing needs, such as the creation of the FHA and public housing.

The Housing Act of 1949 further acknowledged the responsibility of the Federal government in the national housing goal:

> The Congress hereby declares that the general welfare and security of the Nation and the health and living standards of its people require housing production and related community development sufficient to remedy the serious housing shortage, through the clearance of slums and blighted areas, and the realization as soon as feasible of the goal of a decent home and a suitable living environment for every American family, thus contributing to the development of communities and to the advancement of the growth, wealth and security of the Nation. (P.L. 171, the National Housing Act of 1949)

In addition to acknowledging the government's responsibility in housing, the 1949 Housing Act specified the housing problem as a "housing shortage," or supply problem, and thus treated the problem by authorizing 810,000 new public housing units to be constructed over the next six years at a rate of 135,000 units a year (CQ, 1949).

The 1960s marked the beginning of a shift in political ideology, as the problem focused more on income than supply, and ideology of responsibility began to teeter from the state to the individual. The urban renewal and "Great Society" of the 1960s acknowledged the need for the State to become involved in the housing of the American people and thus proposed the rent supplement program to assist individuals relocated by the urban initiatives. The proposal by President Johnson to allow eligible households to rent from the private market (versus the construction of new public housing facilities) initiated the shift from perceiving housing as a supply to seeing it as an income problem. Despite such a proposal, opposition came from Republicans and conservative Democrats who claimed the program would create a socialist environment and American families needed to improve their living accommodations by their own effort (CQ, 1965). The implementation of the subsidized tenant-based housing program in 1974, focusing on the problem of income, was not met with much opposition as the decision was significantly influenced by an economic factor, the then-current housing recession. Thus, Quadrant 4 of Figure 2 depicts the era of the proposal and implementation of subsidized tenant-based housing with the responsibility of the state and the focus on an income problem to adequate housing.

Quadrant 1 of Figure 2 signifies that the federal government views access to adequate housing as a personal responsibility and as a supply problem. Basically, if housing is present, individuals must access housing on their own; if housing is not present, individuals must make other arrangements until housing becomes available. The 1980s marked a rapidly decreasing federal housing budget, and a shift in ideology away from the 1949 national housing goal of state responsibility towards personal responsibility, less government, and deficit reduction at any cost (U.S. House, 1985). During this timeframe, the budget of the subsidized tenant-based housing program, along with the public housing program, was greatly reduced without addressing the consequences of these cuts on individuals and families.

Quadrant 3 of Figure 2 depicts housing policy from the 1990s to the present. During the 1990s, the federal government attempted to revive the federal housing programs by increasing the appropriations to the subsidized tenant-based housing program. A shift away from the federal government's responsibility to personal responsibility remained strong as the goal was to eliminate long-term dependency of recipients and promote strong incentives for recipients to become self-sufficient. In order to demonstrate the ideology of personal responsibility, the Quality Housing and Work Responsibility Act (QHWRA) of 1998 (P.L. 105-276) implemented an eight-hour a month work requirement for recipients of subsidized tenant-based housing (CQ, 1998).

Policy

Written policy specifies the goal(s) of the program and guidelines for implementation, in addition to authorizations and appropriations. The changes that occur in legislation often force changes in implementation. In regard to the Section 8 program, the authors are most interested in the resources, communication, and enforcement that the Section 8 housing program's written policy produces.

Resources

The Section 8 housing program is an intergovernmental program, which can best be described as an inclusive-authority model in which the designation is inclusive; the relationship is dependent, and the authority pattern is hierarchal (Wright, 1982). The implementation of the Section 8 housing program at the local level depends on decisions made by the federal government and the Department of Housing and Urban Development (HUD), which are often reported to PHAs by the local HUD field offices. Consequently, the budget for Section 8 housing is appropriated by Congress to HUD, which is then transferred to the HUD field offices and administered to PHAs. In determining how resources impact the shape and content of the Section 8 housing program, an analysis of authorizations and appropriations are necessary.

Authorizations. In 1999, after four years of no new incremental Section 8 housing units, Congress provided 50,000 new vouchers to be competitively awarded to support families making the transition from welfare to work (HUD, 2000). In 2000, 60,000 units were provided that were not directed to a particular housing purpose or clientele, but rather were competitively awarded to PHAs through a Notice of Funding Availability (NOFA) after funds were first allocated to HUD's field offices through a needs-based fair share formula (HUD, 2000). Additionally 79,000 incremental vouchers were provided in 2001; 25,000 in 2002; and an estimated 34,000 vouchers in 2003 (CQ, 2001; CQ, 2002, Office of Management and Budge [OMB], 2003).

Appropriations. The Section 8 program is a formula-based program where HUD determines how much money is needed annually to properly implement the Section 8 program, and then proposes this figure to Congress. The proposed figure is based on the Annual Contributions Contracts (ACC) submitted by local PHAs, which includes the costs to renew all current housing vouchers, and the administrative fees for the program administered at that particular PHA. The ACC is in effect for 12 months and once approved, determines the amount of funds the PHA will receive throughout the year. The actual appropriations for the Section 8 program has continued to increase each year since 2000, from 4.8 billion dollars, to an estimated 16.4 billion dollars in 2004 (OMB, 2002; OMB, 2004). Budget requests have fluctuated since 2000 from 7.4 billion dollars to 19.9 billion dollars in 2002 to 4.5 billion dollars in 2004 (OMB, 2000; OMB, 2002, OMB, 2004).

The housing policy produces resources, which in turn determines the households served and households not served. In regard to Section 8 housing, there are currently 1.8 million low-income households currently being served through the Section 8 housing voucher program, with 4.8 million total household members (HUD, 2004). Households not served include a significant waiting list across the country with a national average of 11 months (HUD, 2000). New York City and Washington, D.C. average a waiting list of 8 years; Los Angeles, 10 years, and the waiting list in Columbus, Ohio consists of 10,600 eligible individuals with the next available housing unit going to individuals added to the waitlist in October 2001 (HUD, 2000; Columbus Metropolitan Housing Authority [CMHA], 2003). One-third of the allocated 34,000 new housing vouchers approved by Congress in 2003 could be used in Columbus, Ohio alone. Thirty-seven percent of recipients remaining in Section 8 housing stay for 2-5 years, and 21% stay for 5-10 years (HUD, 2004). Due to the length of stay of recipients, the number of new vouchers authorized each year, and the growing numbers on PHAs' waiting lists, the Section 8 housing program will continue to under-serve eligible recipients who are in need of housing assistance.

Communication

The federal regulations (24 CFR 982) serve as a manual to the PHAs detailing the requirements for administering the program, accepting recipients and landlords, and developing the administrative plan. The administrative plan of local PHAs allow the federal government to give some discretion to the PHAs in regard to specific areas, such as selection from the waiting list, and housing quality standards, yet these discretions must be approved by HUD and fall under the broader guidelines of the federal regulations. Communication is two-way from the federal HUD to the local PHAs with the local HUD field offices acting as liaisons. Written documents serve as the main source of communication as the federal HUD communicates through the federal regulations and local PHAs communicate back through the Administrative Plan. Additional on-going communication occurs between local PHAs, HUD field offices, and the federal department of HUD, which often includes acknowledgement of changes in the federal regulations, or recipients' complaints or concerns.

Enforcement

Enforcement of the Section 8 program's rules and regulations are explicitly stated in the CFR, and sanctions and/or incentives are implemented when deemed necessary. The CFR states PHAs "must comply with the consolidated ACC, the application, HUD regulations and other requirements and the PHA Administrative Plan" (24 CFR 982.153). Sanctions will be implemented if PHAs fail to enforce the federal regulations, such as housing quality standards or administrative responsibilities, and can include the reallocation of funds to other PHAs, a reduction of administrative funds, and/or a freeze on withdrawal of funds from the depositary (24 CFR 982.152; 155; 156). Incentives include the ability to apply for additional funds through the Notice of Funding Availability (NOFA) where the PHA's "capacity and capability to administer the program" are taken into consideration (24 CFR 982.104). With enforcement of rules and regulations, implementation of the Section 8 program on a local level can vary across PHAs depending on the presence of sanctions and/or incentives, thus impacting the implementation of the Section 8 program and the service to recipients.

Administrative Skills

The administrative skills of local PHAs can impact the shape and content of the Section 8 housing program administered in the PHA's geographical region. Three areas are identified as potentially impacting the implementation of the Section 8 housing program: (a) Administrative Plan; (b) Section 8 Management Assessment Program (SEMAP); and (c) Notice of Funding Availability (NOFA).

Administrative Plan. The CFR specifies:

> the PHA must adopt a written administrative plan that establishes local policies for administration of the program in accordance with HUD requirements. The administrative plan and any revisions of the plan must be formally adopted by the PHA Board of Commissioners or other authorized HA officials. The administrative plan states PHA policy on matters for which the PHA has discretion to establish local policies. (24 CFR 982.54)

The local PHAs do have authorization to develop agency specific rules and regulations that must be specified in the administrative plan. Such discretion includes selection and admission of applicants, issuing or denying vouchers, occupancy policies, encouraging participation by owners of suitable units located outside areas of low income or minority concentration, how to determine who remains in the program if a family breaks up, informal review and hearing procedures for participants, and housing quality standards inspections (24 CFR 982.54).

Section 8 Management Assessment Program (SEMAP). The administration of the Section 8 housing program is under continual evaluation through the Section 8 Management Assessment Plan (SEMAP).

The CFR states the "PHA must maintain complete and accurate accounts, and other records for the program in accordance with HUD requirements, in a manner that permits a speedy and effective audit" (24 CFR 982.158). From the local PHA's records, SEMAP measures the performance of the PHA in fourteen key areas including selection from the waiting list, rent reasonableness, determination of adjusted income, and housing quality standards enforcement (HUD, 2001). SEMAP assist HUD in monitoring the administration of the PHA and in targeting particular PHAs that need improvement, sanction, and/or incentives.

Notice of Funding Availability (NOFA). HUD notifies local PHAs of a special source of funding though NOFA, which includes funds awarded on a competitive basis. The availability of these special funds assists local PHAs in increasing services to eligible recipients. This special notice informs PHAs of the availability of funds and the requirements in order to apply. The CFR explains the application process for special funding and the requirement of HUD to deem the PHA capable of obtaining the funds and having the capacity to adequately utilize the funds (24 CFR 982.4).

Evaluation

Evaluation acts as a feedback loop in the Section 8 housing program policy process. Evaluation contributed to the development of the Section 8 housing program through the Experimental Housing Allowance Program (EHAP), and continues to impact current and potential future policy decisions through SEMAP, research conducted through HUD's Policy Development and Research (PD&R), and private or contracted researchers from think tanks, universities, and interest groups.

Experimental Housing Allowance Program (EHAP). In the 1970s, Congress instructed HUD to provide, on an experimental basis, low-income families with allowances to enable families to obtain housing of their choice. The EHAP was the first evaluation of the Section 8 housing program and ran from 1971-1980 in twelve locations with nearly 50,000 households (HUD, 2001). Based on this evaluation of the housing allowance program, HUD determined three outcomes: (a) housing stock could be preserved by encouraging owners to repair housing; (b) families were able to move to better neighborhoods; and (c) families were able to pay their share of the rent agreement (HUD, 2001). The combination of the positive preliminary results from EHAP and a severe housing recession lead to the implementation of the Section 8 housing program in 1974 before the full attainment of EHAP findings.

SEMAP. As stated above, SEMAP measures PHA's performance on administering the Section 8 housing program. From the evaluation, HUD utilizes the performance score to monitor PHA's implementation of the Section 8 housing program and intervene when necessary.

Policy Development & Research (PD&R). Congress has continually appropriated funds to the PD&R division of HUD to conduct research on housing related issues. PD&R disseminates research findings through website and journal publications and through congressional testimony. Such an evaluation study includes the Moving to Opportunity (MTO) experimental program examining the economic and social impacts on very poor families who have the chance to move out of subsidized housing in the poorest neighborhoods of five very large American cities; Baltimore, Boston, Chicago, Los Angeles, and New York City (Katz, Kling, & Liebman, 2001). The experiment evaluates three groups: (a) the experimental group consisting of families who receive Section 8 housing vouchers combined with housing counseling; (b) a comparison group who receives Section 8 housing vouchers, but no housing counseling; and (c) a control group consisting of individuals who receive no new housing assistance and no housing counseling (Katz, Kling, & Liebman, 2001). Other published evaluation research by PD&R includes property value impacts of dispersed housing subsidy programs (Galster, Smith, & Tatian, 1999); success rates of housing vouchers (Pistilli, 2001; Finkel & Buron, 2001); and utilization rates of housing vouchers (Finkel et al., 2003).

Through evaluation and research, program administrators, HUD, Congress, and the current political administration, can determine the extent that the Section 8 housing program is meeting the goals stated in the Section 8 housing policy, along with the intended and unintended consequences of the policy and program. Evaluation and research findings can impact future policy, alter the shape and content of the Section 8 housing program, and potentially increase the quality of services to Section 8 housing recipients.

WORKING TO CREATE CHANGE: SOCIAL WORKERS AND THE SECTION 8 POLICY MODEL

For those social workers who work with clients in need of stable housing, the availability of vouchers and eligibility criteria for receiving vouchers can and do impact the ability for practitioners to assist clients in finding affordable, safe, and stable housing. In essence, as Blau and

Abramovitz (2004) have noted of social policy in general, the structure and content of Section 8 housing policy has a direct impact on social work practitioners' ability to successfully intervene with a client in the housing arena. Social policies, including the Section 8 housing program, are not static but are amenable to change. Social workers, with their knowledge of client need and of the impact of social policies on their clients' outcomes, are in a good position to work for change in social policy (Haynes & Mickelson, 1997). Blau and Abramovitz write of the need for social workers to work for change in social policy:

> . . . there is at least one other fact about social welfare policy, if you think that it serves you and your clients poorly, then you should fight to change it. Even if you do not win at first, you may in the future, because the history of social welfare policy shows that change is one of its few constants. (2004, p. 12)

The remainder of this article will focus on how social workers, themselves, can use the proposed Section 8 policy model as a heuristic for understanding where and how to impact Section 8 policy. Selectively drawing from Haynes and Mickelson (1997), we will outline five potential avenues for working for change in the Section 8 housing policy and will link these activities back to the proposed Section 8 policy model.

Monitoring the Policy Process

As Haynes and Mickelson (1997) argue, social workers interested in affecting change in social policies need to monitor the legislative and bureaucratic processes that shape policy. This involves, first and foremost, the need to develop an understanding of how ideas become policies and how these policies are implemented. The policy process is more than just a bill becoming a law; the process also involves fiscal allocations and administrative changes/executive orders that can shape the form and structure of a policy beyond what was in the original legislation. With this basic knowledge in hand, social workers should keep abreast of what policy changes are pending and where these changes are occurring. Such knowledge can aid practitioners in determining where to target their policy change efforts. Those social workers interested in working to change the Section 8 program need to be aware of what and where changes in the policy are taking place if they wish to maximize their policy changing efforts. An example, which will be used throughout the remainder of this paper, is of social service workers at a family service agency who notice an increase in the number of client families who are remaining homeless for long periods of time. In monitoring the bureaucracy, workers at such an agency can determine what changes, if any, are occurring around Section 8 policy. These workers can target their policy changing efforts to those parts of the policy process that are ripe for change.

We suggest that monitoring the legislative and bureaucratic processes that shape Section 8 policy is intimately tied to the entire Section 8 policy model as described above. This model provides a blueprint for following how, where, and under what conditions Section 8 policy changes over time. Through using the entire model as an aid, the social work practitioner can monitor changes in Section 8 policy and determine how and where to intervene.

Collecting and Disseminating Information Around Client Need

A second way in which social workers can impact social policy is to collect and disseminate information on client needs (Haynes & Mickelson, 1997). Social work practitioners and the agencies for which they work are in a unique situation to collect information on client problems and needs. This information can be collected on two levels. First, agencies can collect statistics on client demographics, service use, and service need that can be used to make the case for changes to existing policy. For example, an agency that works with families can track the number of persons who are homeless or at risk of becoming homeless, the amount of time it takes to secure housing for these clients, and the reasons/causes clients give for being homeless or at risk of becoming homeless (e.g., not enough income to support housing or difficulty in locating affordable housing). Such information can be used to argue for expanding the number of vouchers available in a particular location. Second, social workers can collect case illustrations that speak to the need for policy change. When used with statistical information, case illustrations touch persons at an emotional level and provide a human face to statistics. Continuing with the example stated above, a social worker can write a case story of a mother/father struggling to keep her/his family from the streets.

Collecting information is not enough to affect change in social policy. The information also needs to be disseminated to persons in positions to directly impact social policy, such as legislators and program administrators at the local, state, and national levels. The collected information can be disseminated through both testimonials (face-to-face interactions with those in positions to affect change and in public hearings), and written communication (letters, agency newsletters, and agency reports) (Haynes & Mickelson, 1997). As Haynes and Mickelson (1997) point out, clients, too, can be encouraged to take part in the dissemination process. Having clients tell their personal stories puts a human face on the issue.

We see the collection and dissemination of client information as tied to three parts of our Section 8 housing model. First, collection and dissemination of information on client needs can increase an awareness of the economic and social factors that contribute to the further refinement of Section 8 housing policy. Using agency collected information that shows an increased trend in the number of families that are homeless and unable to find housing speaks to underlying social and economic ills that need correction.

Related to increasing awareness of the economic and social factors, collected and disseminated information on the reasons/causes for clients experiencing homelessness or near homelessness can also shape and inform the political debate around the government's role in supporting housing policy, thus having an impact on the political ideology portion of the Section 8 policy model. For example, if clients state that the major reason they are unable to move into housing is the lack of affordable housing, then this information can be used to support interventions supporting increased access to affordable housing. While information about lack of affordable housing as a cause of homelessness or near homelessness may not sway those policy makers with a strong belief in personal responsibility rather than state responsibility for the amelioration of social ills, information on the root causes of homelessness, like the lack of affordable housing, may impact policy makers who are not on the extreme end of the personal reasonability continuum to consider the potential role of government in working to solve this problem.

Finally, the collection and dissemination of information on client needs also speaks to the evaluation component of the Section 8 model. Information collected by agencies can provide information on the effectiveness of meeting the policy's stated goals. Agency-collected information about an increased trend in the number of homeless families who are unable to find affordable housing speaks to a gap between the goal of Section 8 in helping low-income families find a decent place to live and a current lack of affordable, accessible housing. By providing information on either/both social and economic ills and evaluation of program effectiveness, through the use of collection and dissemination of information, the social work practitioner is able to provide to influential persons useful information that can create change in Section 8 policy.

Helping Clients Create Change

A third way in which social worker practitioners can influence policy is through client empowerment and self-determination (Haynes & Mickelson, 1997), both of which are basic tenants of social work practice (Kirst-Ashman & Hull, 2002). Involving clients in affecting change in social policy is a way to achieve client empowerment and self-determination, while still working for change in social policy. One approach to involving clients in policy changing activities is to organize like-minded clients (individuals and/or communities) into client interest groups around a policy issue, such as Section 8. Although the direction and activities of these interest groups should come from the clients, social workers can help by providing technical assistance (e.g., providing them with agency collected information on the scope of the problem, educating them about the policy process, assisting them in developing strategies to influence policy, and connecting them with persons influential in the policy process) and material assistance (e.g., providing a place to meet and access to copy/fax machines).

According to Haynes and Mickelson (1997), another way to work towards client empowerment and self-determination is to encourage clients to vote. This involves both working with clients to register to vote and to ensure that they have the means to vote (e.g., transportation to voting locations). It is important to note that there is federal legislation, the Hatch Act, that limits federal and some state and local officials' involvement in political activities (Haynes & Mickelson, 1997). For example, the Hatch Act allows federal employees to participate in voter registration activities, but prevents them from engaging in voter registration activities that are partisan (U.S. Office of Special Counsel, 2004). In addition, non-governmental social agencies may have guidelines about the role of political activity in the work place. Therefore, it is important that both social work practitioners and the agencies they work for are knowledgeable about the law and that social work providers are knowledgeable about agency policy before engaging in political activities.

The link between client empowerment and self-determination as a method of creating policy change and the Section 8 policy model depends on which empowerment/self-determination activities are being engaged in by both practitioners and clients. The link between organizing clients into client interest groups and the policy model depends on the purpose for which clients are organized. If clients are organized into interest groups to bring awareness of a gap between a current Section 8 policy and the needs of clients, the link is back to social and economic ills and to evaluation. If the goal of the client interest group is more political (e.g., to seek electoral changes at the city, county, state, or federal levels), then the link is to political ideology. These types of groups are seeking to change the political ideology espoused by their representatives at the various levels and branches of government through voting for those elected officials who espouse the clients' political ideology and who view housing issues as the purview of the government and not as an issue of personal responsibility. Likewise, encouraging clients to vote is linked to political ideology.

Social Workers as Administrators

A fourth way that social workers can influence policy is through the role of the social work administrator (Haynes & Mickelson, 1997). Social workers who become administrators are in a unique position to work for changing policy. Social workers who become administrators have an understanding of micro/clinical and macro/political issues and can serve as a bridge between the practice world and the policy world. In addition, social service administrators are often seen as influential members of a community, which can and should facilitate connection and communication with other persons in positions to influence policy, including other social service administrators, local business leaders, and persons in elected office. Using the previous example of a social service agency serving families that has noticed a trend in long term homelessness among served families, social work administrators may use their contacts in the community and their practice experiences to inform and mobilize others in the community to work for change in Section 8 policy. For example, the inability for homeless families to find housing may be linked to a lack of landlords willing to accept Section 8 vouchers. The social work administrator may work with the local housing authority and local landlords to increase the number of available Section 8 units in the community.

The link between social work administrators and the proposed Section 8 policy model is with social and economic ills, evaluation, and administrative skills. In terms of social and economic ills and evaluation, social work administrators are in a position to use their connections to influential members of the community by directly providing information about the gap between current client need and available services. Although the definition of administrative skills mentioned above focuses on the activities of local PHAs and HUD, social work administrators, though their connections with administrators of local PHAs, can also play a role in shaping policy that is in line with our definition of administrative skills. For example, a social service administrator may partner with a local PHA to seek funds from a NOFA or work with landlords to increase the number of housing units that accept Section 8 vouchers. In seeking funds, locating landlords, and collaborating with the local PHA, social service administrators are making an impact in the administrative skills section of the model.

Being a Good Citizen

A final way that social workers can work to change social policy is being a good citizen. Social workers should be involved in the larger political process. One way that social workers can be involved in the political process is to vote in local, state, and federal elections for candidates who support issues and policies that are in line with individual and social work values. In addition to voting for candidates, social workers interested in impacting policy should actively campaign for those candidates (Haynes & Mickelson, 1997). A final way to take an active role in the political process is to run for elected office (Haynes & Mickelson, 1997). According to the National Association of Social Works Political Action for Candidate Election (NASW, PACE, 2003) there are over 150 social workers who hold federal, state, and local offices (NASW, PACE, 2003). It must be noted that the Hatch Act also places some limits on federal, state, and local officials running in partisan elections (U.S. Office of Special Counsel, 2004).

The primary link between being a good citizen and the Section 8 policy model is through political ideology. Political ideology plays a critical role in determining how and if the government chooses to respond to housing issues, including changes that are made to the Section 8 voucher program. One way to create change in political ideology is to vote for or become one of the elected individuals whose responsibility it is to make legislative and executive decisions that impact the course that the Section 8 voucher program will take in the future. In essence, voting for or becoming an elected official can work to change how the government views its role in ameliorating housing ills by potentially moving the solving of the problem toward the responsibility of the government, which may have the effect of strengthening Section 8 policy.

CONCLUSION

Over the course of history, the Section 8 housing program has undergone incremental policy change. The continual policy process of the section 8 housing program can be represented by eight variables that have interacted to affect the shape and content of the housing program. These eight variables include: economic and social factors; political ideologies; policy; resources; communication; enforcement; administrative skills; and evaluation. The combination of these eight variables describe the policy process of the Section 8 housing program, and additionally act as potential avenues of entry by social workers to create future policy change and program implementation.

REFERENCES

Bartelt, D.W. (1993). Housing the "underclass." In M.B. Katz (Ed.), *The "underclass" debate: Views from history* (pp. 135-157). Princeton, NJ: Princeton University Press.

Blau, J., & Abramovitz, M. (2004). *The dynamics of social welfare policy*. New York, N.Y: Oxford University Press.

Congressional Quarterly Almanac. (1949). Congressional Quarterly Service: Washington, DC.

Congressional Quarterly Almanac. (1961). Congressional Quarterly Service: Washington, DC.

Congressional Quarterly Almanac. (1964). Congressional Quarterly Service: Washington, DC.

Congressional Quarterly Almanac. (1965). Congressional Quarterly Service: Washington, DC.

Congressional Quarterly Almanac. (1973). Congressional Quarterly: Washington, DC.

Congressional Quarterly Almanac. (1974). Congressional Quarterly: Washington, DC.

Congressional Quarterly Almanac. (1998). Congressional Quarterly Inc: Washington, DC.

Congressional Quarterly Almanac. (2001). Congressional Quarterly Inc: Washington, DC.

Congressional Quarterly Almanac. (2002). Congressional Quarterly Inc: Washington, DC.

Crane, J. (1991). The epidemic theory of ghettos and neighborhood effects of dropping out and teenage child bearing. *American Journal of Sociology, 96*(5), 1226-1259.

Easton, D. (1965). *A systems analysis of political life*. New York: John Wiley & Sons.

Edelman, M.J. (1971). *Politics as symbolic action: Mass arousal and quiescence*. Chicago: Markham Publishing Company.

Finkel, M., & Buron, L. (2001). *Study on Section 8 voucher success rates: Volume I: Quantitative study of success rates in metropolitan areas*. Washington, DC: U.S. Department of Housing and Urban Development, Office of Policy Development and Research.

Finkel, M., Khadduri, J., Main, V., Pistilli, L., Solari, C., Winkel, K., & Wood, M. (2003). *Costs and utilization in the housing choice voucher program*. Washington, DC: U.S. Department of Housing and Urban Development, Office of Policy Development and Research.

Galster, G., Smith, R.E., & Tatian, P.A. (1999). *Assessing property value impacts of dispersed housing subsidy programs*. Washington, DC: U.S. Department of Housing and Urban Development, Office of Policy Development and Research.

Gotham, K.F., & Wright, J.D. (2000). Housing policy. In J. Midgley, M.B. Tracy, & M. Livermore (Eds.), *The handbook of social policy* (pp. 237-255). Thousand Oaks, CA: Sage Publications, Inc.

Hartung, J.M., & Henig, J.R. (1997). *Housing vouchers and certificates as a vehicle for deconcentrating the poor: Evidence from the Washington, D.C., metropolitan area. Urban Affairs Review, 32*(3), 403-419.

Haynes, K.S., & Mickelson, J.S. (1997). *Affecting change: Social workers in the political arena* (3rd ed.). White Plains, NY: Longman.

Joint Center for Housing Studies of Harvard University (2004). The state of the nation's housing. Retrieved from *http://www.jchs.harvard.edu* on February 24, 2005.

Karger, H.J., & Stoesz, D. (2002). *American social welfare policy: A pluralist approach* (4th ed.). Boston: Allyn and Bacon.

Katz, L.F., Kling, J.R., & Liebman, J.B. (2001). Moving to opportunity in Boston: Early results of a randomized mobility experiment. *The Quarterly Journal of Economics, 116*(2), 607-654.

Kirst-Ashman, K.K., & Hull, G.H., Jr. (2002). *Understanding generalist practice* (3rd ed.). Pacific Groves, CA: Brooks/Cole.

Kleit, R.G. (2001). Neighborhood relations in suburban scattered-site and clustered public housing. *Journal of Urban Affairs*, 22(3), 279-299.

Lindblom, C.E. (1968). *The policy-making process*. Englewood Cliffs, NJ: Prentice-Hall.

Mitchell, J.P. (1985). The historical context for housing policy. In J.P. Mitchell (Ed.), *Federal housing policy & programs* (pp. 3-17). New Brunswick, NJ: Rutgers.

National Association of Social Workers Political Action for Candidate Election (NASW. PACE). (2003). *Demographics of Social Workers in Elected Offices, 2003*. Retrieved September 24, 2004, from http://www.socialworkers.org/pace/characteristics.asp.

Pistilli, L. (2001). *Study on Section 8 voucher success rates: Volume II: Qualitative study of five rural areas*. Washington, DC: U.S. Department of Housing and Urban Development, Office of Policy Development and Research.

U.S. Department of Housing and Urban Development. (2000). *Section 8 tenant-based housing assistance: A look back after 30 years*. Washington, DC: Office of Policy Development and Research.

U.S. Department of Housing and Urban Development. (2001). *Housing choice voucher program guidebook*. Washington, DC.

U.S. Department of Housing and Urban Development, PIH Information Center. (2004). *Resident Characteristic Report*. Retrieved July 23, 2004, from https://pic.hud.gov.

U.S. House. Committee on Banking, Finance, and Urban Affairs. (1974). *Housing in the Seventies.* Washington, DC: Government Printing Office.

U.S. House. Committee on Financial Services. (2003). *Section 8 program housing assistance.* Washington, DC: Government Printing Office.

U.S. House Committee on Banking, Finance, and Urban Affairs. (1985). *Housing Act of 1985, Part 1.* Washington, DC: Government Printing Office.

U.S. Office of Management and Budget. (2000). *Budget of the United States government: Appendix A.* Washington, DC.

U.S. Office of Management and Budget. (2002). *Budget of the United States government: Appendix A.* Washington, DC.

U.S. Office of Management and Budget. (2003). *Budget of the United States government: Appendix A.* Washington, DC.

U.S. Office of Management and Budget. (2004). *Budget of the United States government: Appendix A.* Washington, DC.

U.S. Office of Special Counsel. (2004). *Political Activity (Hatch Act).* Retrieved September 24, 2004, from http://www.osc.gov/hatchact.htm.

U.S. Senate. Committee on Banking, Housing, and Urban Affairs. (1974). *Critique of Housing in the Seventies.* Washington, DC: Government Printing Office.

Wright, D.S. (1982). Models of national/state/local relations. In D.S. Wright (Eds.), *Understanding intergovernmental relations* (pp. 58-66). Monterey, CA: Wadsworth, Inc.

24 CFR 982 (Current through 8/1/04). Text from: *Code of Federal Regulations.* Available from: *LexisNexis* Congressional (Online Service). Bethesda, MD: Congressional Information Service.

Toward a More Inclusive Poverty Knowledge: Traumatological Contributions to the Poverty Discourse

Shawn A. Cassiman

SUMMARY. This paper posits that specialization within disciplines has enabled a fragmentation of knowledge in poverty research, which results in individualistic explanations for poverty that arise naturally from disconnects inherent in isolating frameworks. It proposes that the use of a traumatological framework provides nuances of argument missing from previous discussions, which may allow us to more critically examine the 'culture of poverty' thesis. Such an examination may lead us to consider an alternative explanation. Rather than inherent cultural attributes, descriptors of poverty populations may be manifestations of the symptoms produced by the violence of poverty and other life experiences, and the resultant trauma.

KEYWORDS. Culture, poverty, social work, trauma, violence

Shawn A. Cassiman is affiliated with the School of Social Work, University of Wisconsin-Madison, 1350 University Avenue, Madison, WI 53706.

[Haworth co-indexing entry note]: "Toward a More Inclusive Poverty Knowledge: Traumatological Contributions to the Poverty Discourse." Cassiman, Shawn A. Co-published simultaneously in *The Social Policy Journal* (The Haworth Press, Inc.) Vol. 4, No. 3/4, 2005, pp. 93-106; and: *Cutting-Edge Social Policy Research* (ed: Richard Hoefer) The Haworth Press, Inc., 2005, pp. 93-106. Single or multiple copies of this article are available for a fee from The Haworth Document Delivery Service [1-800-HAWORTH, 9:00 a.m. - 5:00 p.m. (EST). E-mail address: docdelivery@ haworthpress.com].

Available online at http://www.haworthpress.com/web/SPJ

doi:10.1300/J185v04n03_06

INTRODUCTION

The goals of this paper are: (1) to emphasize the necessity of an inclusive poverty discourse, (2) to demonstrate how uniquely capable and potentially culpable the discipline of social work may be in formulating the poverty policy debate, and (3) to demonstrate how the inclusion of knowledge of trauma experience may be relevant to poverty research and enriching to the discourse. Most specifically, this paper draws upon work on trauma by Kira (2001), which focuses upon historical trauma and its implications. As an example of inclusive poverty research this paper holds as a fundamental assumption that the breadth of knowledge extent within the social work profession is applicabile to social policy. The conclusion this paper articulates is one that shifts the emphasis from a culture of poverty as proposed by Lewis (1969) to a dominant culture's participation in the business of manufacturing poverty through social policy design and poverty discourse, resulting in a traumatized citizenry. In other words, populations previously vilified for their deviant natures may be viewed, instead, through a lens that focuses upon their trauma symptoms. This shift in focus may invite us to draw different conclusions as to why many anti-poverty policies have been ineffectual and may lead to the assumption that only multi-level and universal social welfare programs will have any lasting impact upon poverty and inequality. Much like the function of a systems perspective in practice, the inclusion of trauma in discussions of poverty policy broadens the framework.

HISTORY

Specialization is not peculiar to social work but is evident in most social science disciplines (O'Connor, 2001). Neither is specialization particularly negative, as specialization within social work has contributed to a wealth of knowledge within specific fields or subfields, such as gerontology, trauma, mental health and substance abuse. However, such specialization may lead to an exclusive relationship with social welfare policy, in which specialists approach policy only in terms of their field of practice. Specialization may contribute to the dichotomy between policy and practice and the tension between professionalism and activism rooted in the history of social work (Ehrenreich, 1985; Katz, 1989; Reisch & Andrews, 2002). In fact, the impetus for specialization may arise, in part, from the desire for professional recognition. It may also arise in a desire to advance the need for recognition of the population of interest.

Such specialization within disciplines has contributed to a fragmentation of knowledge in poverty research that results in individualistic explanations for poverty that lead to disconnects inherent in isolating frameworks. For instance, discussions of culture in social work have most frequently centered upon issues of practice rather than issues of policy. This is the case, it is argued, because historically " In matters relating to poverty, social work conceded the field of quantitative analysis to social scientists, primarily economists" (Stoesz, 1999, p. 189). It is also the case that the cultural discourse is rarely critical of the *dominant* culture. Such a critique is missing from social policy discourse, largely because theoretical models are based on econometrics that provide limited opportunity for self-critique. Sackrey and Schneider (2002) articulate this lack as a result of neo-classical economists' benign views of capitalism and their perception of themselves as "dispassionate experts."

In other words, social work's concession of (or exclusion from) the poverty policy debate, and mainstream poverty research's consistent neglect of a broader cultural critique, ensures that any discussion of race, gender or class, leads *logically,* to individual deficit discussions, considerations of the 'underclass' and 'culture of poverty' type theses, for no other explanations fit rationally within such models.

CULTURE AND SOCIAL WORK

The cultural discourse within social work has experienced a variety of interpretations in its evolution toward the multiculturalism we are most familiar with today. Curran (2003) documents the significance of the cultural discourse in post-war social work, and its many incarnations as relativist, paternalistic or deterministic. This discourse additionally almost always occurs within a psychological context. This union of psychology and culture lies at the root of Oscar Lewis' (1969) "culture of poverty" thesis. This thesis came to fruition in Murray's (1984) *Losing Ground*, in which ideations of 'intergenerational transmission,' 'dependency,' and 'inability to defer gratification' in combination with rational choice discussions, became the basis of welfare reform arguments.

Central to Murray's (1984) argument and since adopted in mainstream policy discourse is the 'generosity' of welfare benefits and its effect on the incentives to work. In fact, rather than generous, the welfare benefits in the U.S. are minimal in comparison to other developed nations (Rank & Hirschl, 2002). Furthermore, using Sweden's welfare state as a comparison, generous welfare benefits do not necessarily correlate with decreased work participation (Sackrey, Schneider, & Knoedler, 2002).

For the sake of discussion, let us accept the possibility that people experiencing poverty do indeed exhibit those tendencies described above, i.e., inability to defer gratification, or present oriented lifestyles, 'dependency,' and the cultural transmission of poverty across generations. Putting aside for the most part the issue of dependency in this paper, I will instead focus upon deferment of gratification and intergenerational transmission of poverty, and the question of how such descriptors are commonly used when documenting the symptoms experienced by trauma victims.

THE EFFECTS OF POVERTY AND STRUCTURAL VIOLENCE

Social science scholars have provided extensive documentation of the lasting impact of poverty and inequality. For instance, Smeeding (1997) cites several medical journal articles that report, " . . . high and increasing economic inequality is highly correlated with high and increasing mortality" (p. 4). We are all aware of the impact of hunger on school performance, of impoverished schools on academic outcomes, lack of affordable housing in combination with low-wage jobs and homelessness, and so on. In spite of our awareness, what has been largely missing from the discourse to date is the violent nature of the poverty experience.

Typically, when we consider violence in a context of poverty, we think of violent communities, gang, and drug related violence. While obvious examples of violent aspects of the poverty experience exist, we remain relatively oblivious to more subtle examples. Traditional conceptualizations of violence focus primarily on interpersonal physical violence and frequently ignore institutional, structural, and psychological forms of violence. A broader and more inclusive conceptual framework is proposed by scholars (Iadicola & Shupe, 2003) of the sociology of violence, with violence being defined as ". . . any action or structural arrangement that results in physical or nonphysical harm to one or more persons" (p. 23). Such a conceptualization of violence is inclusive of actions not only on the part of individuals, but includes violence that is institutional and structural in nature. In addition, the authors emphasize that intent is not an issue in the perpetration of violence. Furthermore, neither the perpetrator nor the victim of violence need be aware of the violent nature of the act.

The scholarly literature that comes closest to capturing the violent, painful and debilitating nature of poverty is comprised primarily of qualitative studies of poverty populations. In *Tell Them Who I Am*, the recounting of the lives of homeless women in Washington, D.C., Liebow (1993) documents the women's struggles for the simplest of things, such as water, sleep, and relative safety. Stress, powerlessness, desperation, and fear run like a common thread through all their lives. *Lives on the Edge* is a qualitative account of the experiences of poor children, further marginalized and traumatized by an educational system designed for an "at risk" population (Polakow, 1993). In 1982 Deborah Belle published her account of poor single mothers in which she draws the conclusion, "The long-term problems of poverty, burdensome responsibilities, and foreclosed opportunity contribute more heavily to the depression of low-income mothers, than a single crisis or traumatic event" (p. 81).

"*So You Think I Drive a Cadillac*?" (Seccombe, 1999) consists of interviews with women on welfare in the wake of welfare reform. In the course of listening and telling the stories of these women, the author describes the phenomena of attribution among welfare recipients. When describing other recipients, the women frequently used individual explanatory frameworks for welfare receipt (laziness, lack of ambition, etc.). When explaining their own receipt, however, structural problems were the focus. This explanatory framework speaks to the power of the welfare queen myth and its impact upon recipients. Whether working poor or welfare poor (and the two are not mutually exclusive), adult or child, this body of research is illustrative of hooks' (2000) observation, "To be poor in the United States today is to be always at risk, the object of scorn and shame" (p. 45).

THE TRAUMA PARADIGM

The trauma paradigm is not without its critics. Summerfield's (2001) critique of the trauma paradigm and particularly Post Traumatic Stress Disorder (PTSD) seems to be focused on either its broad usefulness or its misuse. For instance, in describing the usefulness of the trauma paradigm to humanitarian programs, he states that it is often used as,

". . . a basis for capturing and addressing the impact of events like war . . ." (p. 95). He worries, however, that the Western nature of the paradigm limits its usefulness in non-Western locations. While I applaud attention to the subject of location, it seems this critique assumes hegemony of Western identity only in discussions of the trauma paradigm. For instance, we (Westerners) seem to be much less prone to such self-critique when transferring Western theories of development. In order to be applicable to other cultural and ethnic groups and situations, social work finds the need to constantly reevaluate theories and theoretical implications of positionality, whether those positions include the historical, cultural, class or gender positions. We will notice the usefulness of Kira's (2001) framework as demonstrated by the way in which he prioritizes positionality and history.

However, Summerfield's (2001) critique is also concerned with the trivialization of trauma, a very legitimate concern. He states, "In Western societies the conflation of distress with 'trauma' increasingly has a naturalistic feel; it has become part of everyday descriptions of life's vicissitudes" (p. 96). While I agree that we must be careful not to overgeneralize and so trivialize the trauma experience, it seems this statement is rather too simplistic and may allude to the privileged position of the speaker. For instance, a car that won't start is a minor irritant to an individual with sufficient resources to consider it so. However, a car that won't start could be one of many stressors of the week for an individual with few financial or human resources. It could also lead to the loss of a job, as many low-wage jobs provide little security, which could lead to the loss of housing, and so on. Or, we can consider a common but chronic illness: to an individual with health insurance and employment benefits that support an employee in illness, this could be an irritating inconvenience, but to an individual with no insurance and no employee benefits, the situation may have far greater consequences. In combination with other stressors or in combination with a history of trauma, we might well argue that this is an example of the trauma experience. Obviously the nature of stress and trauma are relative and what is considered a trivial inconvenience to one person may have a devastating impact upon another.

Furedi (2000; 2004) offers a similar critique of what he calls the "therapy culture." However, while Summerfield (2001) supposes the individual motive for seeking the PTSD label to be the legitimization of a claim for redress or action (which he finds problematic), Furedi argues that the therapy culture is imposed upon the individual, which robs them of the ability to cope. While there are times such a critique would be useful, when analyzing the dependency narrative for instance, it seems evident that the critique is not a useful one when discussing Kira's (2001) taxonomy. Rather, it appears as if Furedi's critique of the therapy culture is most concerned with the marketing of clienthood as problematic, while Kira's taxonomy illustrates the potential impacts of failure to interrogate poverty policy. In fact, since the trauma paradigm does reveal avenues for claims and demands, perhaps Ferudi would agree with Gilfus (1999) about the necessity of the politicization of the trauma paradigm, as he has obviously politicized the "therapy culture." Fortunately, we will see that Kira's (2001) taxonomy allows us to capture some of the nuance of experience and the ways in which history and experience may add to or build the layers of risk in the exposure to trauma.

Like Summerfield, Gilfus (1999) asserts that ". . . trauma theory has rapidly become a dominant psychological paradigm of our time . . ." (p. 1239). While recognizing the value of trauma paradigms, Gilfus is able to articulate a weakness within trauma theory: "Mainstream trauma research and practice, however, tend to be more medicalized and less political" (p. 1241). In an effort to instigate movement from the medical to the political, it is imperative that we shift the discourse of trauma from the purely individualistic toward a trauma discourse inclusive of the societal and structural.

For instance, by ignoring the "inequalities of power relations" in other realms of society, we also ignore the ways in which people experience trauma on multiple levels and in multiple locations. According to Gilfus (1999), this precludes us from ". . . being able to see *contexts of oppression and differentially distributed vulnerability to traumatic injury and the damages caused by obscuring those contexts* [emphasis added]" (p. 1249).

Research on the taxonomy of trauma (Kira, 2001) leads to a much broader and more inclusive conceptualization of trauma. These taxonomies of trauma serve to organize trauma into categories and layers of experience often missing from mainstream trauma paradigms. Kira organized trauma into two distinct classifications: (1) ". . . according to impact upon different areas of individual functioning" (p. 75), and (2) ". . . based on the objective or external characteristics of the traumatic event" (p. 78). Levels of functioning include attachment, autonomy/identity/individuation, interdependence or disconnectedness, achievement/ self-actualization, and survival. Much of the discussion of impact upon levels of functioning focuses upon psychological theories of a just world, in which an individual's sense of safety and basic assumptions of deservedness are shattered by trauma (Gilfus, 1999). By pointing out differences in worldviews between racial and ethnic minorities, poor and working-class people, Gilfus demonstrates, "The current paradigm in trauma treatment and research is culturally bound, reflecting a White, middle-class, never-victimized worldview" (p. 1251). Adelman (2003) describes the problem as one in which ". . . majority group members control the interpretation of what it means to take culture into account" (p. 113). In other words, individuals are informed of what is or is not traumatic, what it means to take culture into account, and schooled in "the just world" whether or not their lived experiences confirm the normative discourse.

This worldview and the interpretation of culture are relevant to the second set of classifications used by Kira (2001). These external characteristics of trauma classifications are further explained in categories of external and internal.

> Traumatogenic stimuli can be either internally induced, e.g., terminal illness, limb amputation, uncontrollable pain, panic attacks, or externally induced. Externally induced traumatogenic stimuli can be either nature-made, e.g., hurricanes, or man-made. Man-made traumatogenic stimuli can be either person-made (direct trauma) or society-made (indirect trauma transmission). (p. 78)

Kira's (2001) classifications are further refined by assessments of single event or Type I trauma, complex or Type II trauma and sequence of trauma or Type III trauma. Type III trauma is described as having usually accumulative effects, and can "take different sequences in each area of functioning" (p. 78). Additional divisions of society-made trauma occur at the levels of transmission.

Of most relevance to this discussion are complex trauma and type III trauma and the transmission of each, either cross-generationally or historically. Type II is a sequential experience of trauma. Such "ongoing chronic traumatic conditions" have most commonly been associated with physical or sexual abuse and war. Broader, more inclusive conceptions, include poverty, hunger, and illness (p. 82). Closer examination of collective cross-generational trauma transmission includes both historical trauma (such as slavery, for African Americans or genocide for Native Americans or the Jewish experience of the Holocaust) that is inflicted upon a group, and affects the group identity. Historical trauma may in fact be a much more relevant determinant of group experience, particularly when considering the culture of poverty thesis. The research also indicates that historical trauma may affect individuals' response to new trauma. For instance, Native Americans experienced longer lasting PTSD symptoms following service in Vietnam compared to their White counterparts.

Kira (2001) describes the second kind of cross-generational transmission of trauma as the "multi-generational transmission of structural violence that constitutes extreme social disparities" (p. 80). Kira describes such disparities:

> The effects of the structure or social violence created by generating deprived social structures or classes are traumatic to the parents and their children. Poverty, biologically induced traumas such as hunger or prolonged malnutrition, inadequate and crowded shelter, inadequate medical care, unemployment, underemployment or employment in temporary jobs without fringe benefits, all of those cause severe consequences. (p. 81)

Acknowledging such disparities leads to what Gilfus (1999) describes as, ". . . knowledge of 'no just world' or, 'the search for an understanding of the social and political world in which such injustice can occur'" (p. 1252).

This search for understanding occurs at multiple points. Research by Soss (2005) describes the effects upon citizenship and participation as an outcome of experience of such systems. Soss compares the experience of Social Security Disability Insurance (SSDI) claimants with that of the former system of welfare provision, Aid to Families with Dependent Children (AFDC). His research concluded that SSDI recipients felt their claims on the system legitimate, while AFDC recipients experienced their claims as suspect and contingent. These distinct categorical representations of deserving populations versus undeserving populations led to a cohesive group identity in the SSDI (deserving) population. The AFDC (undeserving) population instead experienced a fragmented non-group identity in which each became the deserving exception, and attempted to distance themselves from the undeserving general population. Individuals generalized their experience with the social welfare system to their larger expectations of government representation. As might be predicted, SSDI recipients felt empowered as citizens, while AFDC recipients felt powerless. Schneider and Ingram (1997) articulate the diversity of possible policy experiences,

> Policy designs reflect the social constructions of knowledge, target populations, power relationships, and institutions in the context from which they emerge, and these are conveyed to citizens through the messages, interpretations, and experiences that people have with public policy. (p. 5)

Inclusion of a traumatological framework serves to broaden the cultural critique and leads toward recognition of the role poverty policy, specifically, and social welfare policy design, implementation and discourse, more generally, plays in the health and well-being of citizens. Minimalist policies based on means testing, and focused on often stigmatized populations (in terms of their deservedness), may lead to the production of the very social "ills" we seek to alleviate. Furthermore, politicians and policy makers who design or condone policies that perpetuate high levels of poverty and inequality are complicit in the traumatization of citizens they are charged to serve.

POVERTY AND THE LIFE COURSE

Due in large part to the particularizing of poverty populations, with the focus upon the "underclass" and the "welfare dependent" in media coverage of social policy (Gilens, 1999), many individuals are under the impression that only a small percentage of U.S. citizens will have need to access means tested programs, such as TANF, Food Stamps, SSI, or Medicaid (traditionally conceptualized as 'welfare' programs while excluding other less stigmatized social welfare programs from conceptualizations of welfare). However, research by Rank (2004) dispels such misconceptions and raises our awareness of the actual incidence of welfare use among the U.S. population over the life course: ". . . two-thirds of all Americans between the ages of twenty and sixty-five at some point turn to a public assistance program, while 40 percent of the population access a welfare program in five or more years during their adulthood" (p. 106).

These are startling statistics for three reasons. First, because the awareness that a *majority* of Americans may access means-tested welfare programs over the life course serves to demonstrate the weakness of the arguments (cultural, individualistic) used to define deserving and undeserving poor populations. We must abandon our views of deservingness, unless, as Rank (2004) notes, ". . . we are willing to argue that the majority of us are undeserving . . ." (p. 107). Second, if we must make arguments for universal social welfare policies on the basis of self-interest (which I am unconvinced we must), there is no clearer argument for self-interest than the recognition that the majority of us will have experience with such stigmatizing programs and the implications of such an experience. The final reason is how such an awareness might touch upon all areas of social work practice and influence what Jansson (2003) describes as "policy advocacy." If we use a broader framework, with trauma prevention as the boundaries, we are able to see how each discipline or specialty is impacted in similar ways. This might lead to cross-specialization coalitions that are able to combine resources and expertise for shared policy goals that demonstrate the essential nature of a structural critique.

IMPLICATIONS OF AN INCLUSIVE POVERTY KNOWLEDGE

An examination of social welfare policy in the context of an inclusive poverty knowledge, a knowledge that includes a recognition of the likelihood or susceptibility of the experience of poverty over the life course, an awareness of the violent nature of the poverty experience and the fundamentally traumatic nature of violence, leads us to articulate the need for universal social welfare programs that are preventative rather than corrective. It also shifts the discourse from one of "the poor" to one of poverty. The policy design process informed by such awareness might look much different. How might such policy look? Perhaps much like Social Security or Head Start programs that have been developed due to an awareness of the limitations of a neoclassical economic system reliant upon cheap labor and a "natural" unemployment rate of about 5 percent. It might look very much like the translation of the systems perspective, so useful in practice, to a policy framework.

Abramovitz (2001) reminds us that everyone benefits from social welfare policies. Furthermore, successful challenges of the legitimacy of one system of welfare, such as AFDC, may lead to challenges of other programs, such as Social Security. In addition, scholars (Radcliff, Best, Cushow, & Krueger, 2000) have demonstrated that all citizens are impacted by social welfare policy design. Measuring life satisfaction based upon welfare regime using Epsing-Anderson's (1990) conceptualizations of Liberal (residual-least generous), Corporatist (more generous) and Social Democratic (universal-most generous) the authors found that generous welfare regimes correlated to greater life satisfaction. These results seem to indicate, that even if unable to articulate the importance of the welfare state in their lives, individuals are nevertheless aware of its impact.

An inclusive poverty knowledge is by necessity a knowledge informed by social workers and social work practice. One hallmark of social work is its commitment to social justice. Our history charges us with advocacy not only at the individual level, but also at the policy level. Rather than aspire to be the impersonal expert, social workers must repeat to policy makers that policy is personal. Or as Schram (2002) reminds us, that ". . . the facts are always value-laden, that facts and values cannot be separated, and that attempts to do so will only result in the insidious effects of allowing biases to work their way into ostensibly objective analyses without challenge" (p. 127).

In addition, we need to remember that "reconstructed poverty knowledge would acknowledge and embrace its inherently political nature . . ." (O'Connor, 2001, p. 272). Policy is political insomuch as it defines who has access to the political arena and whose opinions and claims are legitimate (Schram & Soss, 2001; Soss, 1999). As such, policy research should not ascribe to an ideal of apolitical neutrality. When policy discussions are limited to what is considered 'policy relevant,' it falls upon social workers to demonstrate that issues of social justice and basic human rights are more than relevant, and are in fact the very essence of social welfare.

CONCLUSION

Particularizing 'the poor' in tandem with professional specialization, in a context bereft of structural critique, has resulted in the perpetuation of the culture of poverty thesis. While many progressive social work scholars are somewhat reluctant to re-visit issues of pathology and the relationship to 'the poor,' this proposed line of research appears to be timely and of the utmost urgency. As Kira (2001) reminds us, "The direct and indirect cross-generational consequences of such structural violence (poverty and inequality) are devastating and enduring. They can transmit this kind of traumatic conditions across generations" (p. 81). The sooner we recognize the violent nature of poverty and the resultant trauma to those individuals that experience poverty, the sooner we may implement policy interventions to eliminate chronic societally-created structural violence and its effects on future generations.

We must also remind ourselves that avoiding culture of poverty arguments has done little to change the terms of debate, but rather conceded the terrain to conservative policy interests. An awareness of the traumatizing nature of the poverty experience lifts the onus of the culture of poverty from the individual and places it directly upon policy makers and society.

REFERENCES

Abramovitz, M. (2001). Everyone is still on welfare: The role of redistribution in social policy. *Social Work, 46*(4), 297-308.

Adelman, M., Erez, E., & Shalhoub-Kevorkian, N. (2003). Policing violence against minority women in multicultural societies: "Community" and the politics of exclusion. *Police and Society* (7), 103-131.

Belle, D. (Ed.). (1982). *Lives in stress: Women and depression.* Beverly Hills: Sage.

Curran, L. (2003). The culture of race, class, and poverty: The emergence of a cultural discourse in early cold war social work (1946-1963). *Journal of Sociology & Social Welfare, 30*(3), 15-38.

Ehrenreich, J. H. (1985). *The altruistic imagination: A history of social work and social policy in the United States.* London: Cornell University Press.

Epsing-Anderson, G. (1990). *The three worlds of welfare capitalism.* Princeton: Princeton University Press.

Ferudi, F. (2004). Reflections on the medicalization of social experience. *British Journal of Guidance and Counseling*, 32, (3), 413-415.

Ferudi, F. (2003). *Therapy culture: Cultivating vulnerability in an uncertain age.* New York: Routledge.

Gilfus, M. E. (1999). The price of the ticket: A survivor-centered appraisal of trauma theory. *Violence Against Women, 5*(11), 1238-1257.

Gilens, M. (1999). *Why Americans hate welfare: Race, media, and the politics of anti-poverty policy.* Chicago: University of Chicago Press.

hooks, b. (2000). *Where we stand: Class matters.* New York: Routledge.

Iadicola, P., & Shupe, A. (2003). *Violence, inequality, and human freedom* (2nd ed.). Lanham: Rowan & Littlefield Publishers.

Jansson, B. S. (2003). *Becoming an effective policy advocate: From policy practice to social justice* (4th ed.). Pacific Grove: Thomson.

Katz, M. (1989). *The undeserving poor: From the war on poverty to the war on welfare.* New York: Pantheon Books.

Kira, I. A. (2001). Taxonomy of trauma and trauma assessment. *Traumatology, 7*(2), 73-86.

Lewis, O. (1969). The culture of poverty. In Moynihan, D. P. (Ed.), *On understanding poverty: Perspectives from the social sciences.* New York: Basic Books.

Liebow, E. (1993). *Tell them who I am: The lives of homeless women.* New York: Penguin Books.

Murray, C. (1984). *Losing ground: American social policy, 1950-1980.* New York: Basic Books.

O'Connor, A. (2001). *Poverty knowledge: Social science, social policy, and the poor in Twentieth-Century U.S. history.* Princeton: Princeton University Press.

Polakow, V. (1993). *Lives on the edge: Single mothers and their children in the other America*. Chicago: The University of Chicago Press.

Radcliff, B., Best, S., Cushow, S., & Krueger, B. (2000, April 10-13). *Politics, markets, and life satisfaction: The political economy of human happiness in the industrial democracies*. Paper presented at the Political Studies Association-UK, 50th Annual Conference, London.

Rank, M. R. (2004). *One nation underprivileged: Why American poverty affects us all*. Oxford: Oxford University Press.

Rank, M. R., & Hirschl, T. A. (2002). Welfare use as a life course event: Toward a new understanding of the U.S. safety net. *Social Work 47*(3), 237-248.

Reisch, M., & Andrews, J. (2002). *The road not taken: A history of radical social work in the United States*. New York: Brunner-Routledge.

Sackrey, C., Schneider, G., & Knoedler, J. (2002). *Introduction to political economy* (3rd ed.). Cambridge: Economic Affairs Bureau, Inc.

Schneider, A. L., & Ingram, H. (1997). *Policy design for democracy*. Lawrence: University of Kansas Press.

Schram, S. F. (2002). *Praxis for the poor: Piven and Cloward and the future of social science in social welfare*. New York: New York University Press.

Schram, S. F., & Soss, J. (2001). Success stories: Welfare reform, policy discourse, and the politics of research. *The Annals of the American Academy of Political and Social Science, 577*(1), 49-65.

Seccombe, K. (1999). *"So you think I drive a Cadillac?": Welfare recipients' perspectives on the system and its reform*. Boston: Allyn and Bacon.

Smeeding, T. M. (1997, April). *American income inequality in a cross-national perspective: Why are we so different?* Paper presented at the National Policy Association's Conference on "The Growth of Income Disparity," Maxwell School of Citizenship and Public Affairs Syracuse, New York.

Soss, J. (1999). Welfare application encounters: Subordination, satisfaction, and the puzzle of client evaluations. *Administration & Society, 31*(1), 50-94.

Soss, J. (2005). Making clients and citizens: Welfare policy as a source of status, belief, and action. In A. L. I. Schneider, Helen (Ed.), *Deserving and entitled: Social constructions and public policy*. New York: State University of New York Press.

Stoesz, D. (1999). Ideological nostalgia, intellectual narcosis. In G. R. Lowe & Reid, N. P. (Eds.), *The professionalization of poverty: Social work and the poor in the Twentieth century* (pp. 141-160). New York: Aldine De Gruyter.

Summerfield, D. (2001). The invention of post-traumatic stress disorder and the social usefulness of a psychiatric category. *British Medical Journal*, 322, 95-98.

Effects of Work Incentive Policies and Determinants of the Socioeconomic Status of Welfare Leavers in an Economically Disadvantaged Area

Kyoung Hag Lee

SUMMARY. This study explores how work incentive policies influence the socioeconomic status of welfare leavers. Logistic and ordinal regression methods were used to analyze 1999 statewide survey data on West Virginia WORKS leavers. This study found that people who had more months of eligibility remaining for TANF were more likely to have jobs than those with fewer months of eligibility. People who had been sanctioned for noncompliance with work requirements were less likely to have jobs than those who had not been sanctioned. However, childcare assistance had a significant influence on the employment of welfare leavers.

Kyoung Hag Lee, PhD, is affiliated with the Division of Social Work, West Virginia University, Morgantown, WV 26506 (E-mail: leeclark24@hotmail.com).

The author would like to thank Eleanor H. Blakely, Dong Pil Yoon, Barry L. Locke, Ginny V. Majewski of the West Virginia University Division of Social Work for helpful comments and supports, and Karen Harper-Dorton, Director of the Beatrice Ruth Burgess Center in the Division of Social Work at West Virginia University that sponsored this research. The views expressed herein are those of the author, and do not represent the positions of the Beatrice Ruth Burgess Center or the State of West Virginia.

Prepared and presented at the Policy Conference, Charleston, SC, August 7-10, 2004.

[Haworth co-indexing entry note]: "Effects of Work Incentive Policies and Determinants of the Socioeconomic Status of Welfare Leavers in an Economically Disadvantaged Area." Lee, Kyoung Hag. Co-published simultaneously in *The Social Policy Journal* (The Haworth Press, Inc.) Vol. 4, No. 3/4, 2005, pp. 107-125; and: *Cutting-Edge Social Policy Research* (ed: Richard Hoefer) The Haworth Press, Inc., 2005, pp. 107-125. Single or multiple copies of this article are available for a fee from The Haworth Document Delivery Service [1-800-HAWORTH, 9:00 a.m. - 5:00 p.m. (EST). E-mail address: docdelivery@haworthpress.com].

Available online at http://www.haworthpress.com/web/SPJ

doi:10.1300/J185v04n03_07

EITC was significantly associated with the expectation of high economic status. Policy implications are discussed.

KEYWORDS. Welfare reform, work incentive policies, lifetime limits, sanctions, welfare leavers

INTRODUCTION

The Personal Responsibility and Work Opportunity Reconciliation Act (PRWORA) of 1996 replaced the 61-year-old Aid to Families with Dependent Children (AFDC) program with the Temporary Assistance to Needy Families (TANF) program. It also eliminated the program's open-ended entitlement status, provided fixed funding amounts to each state, limited assistance to a maximum of 60 months, and imposed workforce participation rules on states (Karger & Stoesz, 2002).

TANF's main goal was to increase the self-sufficiency of welfare recipients by imposing work incentive policies (GAO, 1999). Non-financial work incentive policies such as lifetime limits on welfare benefits and sanctions for noncompliance with work requirements have played key roles in moving single mothers from welfare to work (Coe, Acs, Lerman, & Watson, 1998). In the past, states had little incentive to remove welfare recipients from programs because fewer recipients meant less federal funding. However, after welfare reform, if states continually failed to meet the mandatory work participation rates, they were subject to the forfeiture of up to a maximum of 21 percent of the federal funding (Dilger, 2004). States imposed strict lifetime limits and sanctions to increase work participation. Also, financial work incentive policies (e.g., Medicaid, food stamps, and so on) were important factors for supporting welfare recipients in leaving welfare with jobs (Cancian & Meyer, 2000).

Since welfare reform in 1996, there has been a radical reduction in the caseload of welfare recipients and a dramatic increase in work participation. In Fiscal Year 2001, the number of average monthly TANF recipients was 57 percent lower than the average monthly number of AFDC recipients in Fiscal Year 1996 (DHHS, 2000). In Fiscal Year 2000, 33 percent of adult welfare recipients were working–a three-fold increase since Fiscal Year 1996. However, studies on welfare leavers have argued that many people who left welfare did not work continually and their earnings were very low; moreover, they faced economic hardships (Plein, 2001).

In the literature of welfare reform, numerous studies have explored factors that influence welfare recipients in their efforts to successfully stay off welfare with stable jobs and high income (Sandefur & Cook, 1998). Some studies examined factors that influence the unemployment and economic problems of welfare leavers or factors that induce welfare leavers to return to welfare with the problems of employment and economic well-being (Lieberman & Mancuso, 2001). Other studies explored the effects of the work incentive policies of some states on the lives of former welfare recipients (Pavetti & Bloom, 2001; Coe et al., 1998).

However, little is known about how the work incentive policies of a rural Appalachian state have influenced the socioeconomic status of people who left welfare after the 1996 welfare reform. This study makes a unique contribution to the growing body of literature on welfare reform by examining the relationship between work incentive policies and the socioeconomic status of welfare leavers in West Virginia, an economically disadvantaged state with the fifth highest poverty rate in the nation (U.S. Census Bureau, 2003). Studying the effects of work incentive policies in such an environment is quite important because the majority of studies have focused on low-income families in urban areas. By exploring the socioeconomic status of former welfare recipients, this research provides a case study of the potential consequences of work incentive policies in a state with a long-term history of economic recession.

WELFARE REFORM IN WEST VIRGINIA

When President Clinton signed the PRWORA of 1996, West Virginia already had a welfare reform plan called WV WORKS. WV WORKS was implemented on a county-by-county basis through the latter part of 1997, switching to an across-the-state basis by early 1998 (Dilger, 2004). The program was a work first program that emphasized the self-sufficiency of welfare recipients by imposing mandatory work requirements.

In order to avoid financial penalties from the federal government, decision makers in West Virginia pursued a policy of radical case closure to meet the new requirements for caseload reduction credit (Plein, 2001). Between January 1997 and June 1999, caseloads were dramatically reduced in West Virginia, with 68.5 percent of welfare recipients (67,658 out of 98,680) leaving the welfare program compared with the reduction of 39.7 percent of the national welfare caseload (4.5 million out of 11.4 million) (DHHS, 2000).

However, even though most policy makers believed that welfare reform was working because of the reductions, fewer than one-third of former welfare recipients were finding jobs (Fisher, 1998). Thus, it is important to explore how work incentive policies influence success in exiting the welfare system, along with the employment, and economic status of former welfare recipients in economically disadvantaged areas.

LITERATURE REVIEW

Important Factors Affecting the Socioeconomic Status of Welfare Leavers

Considerable research has documented that educational attainment and participation in job training were significantly associated with increasing the employment and income of welfare leavers (Tweedie, Reichert, & O'Connor, 1999; Vartanian & McNamara, 2000). Former welfare recipients who had a physical or psychological disability were less likely than people without a disability to increase their employment and economic well-being (Danziger & Seefeldt, 2002).

Numerous studies have documented the impact of marriage on self-sufficiency, indicating that welfare recipients who were married were more likely to permanently leave welfare and to have a higher income (Sandefur & Cook, 1998; Vartanian & McNamara, 2000). Between 1996 and 2000, nationwide, the caseloads of black families have fallen more rapidly than the caseloads of white families (Finegold & Staveteig, 2002). Black welfare leavers have been employed more than whites between 1997 and 1999. However, the median wage of black welfare leavers was $6.88, compared with $7.31 for white welfare leavers (Finegold & Staveteig, 2002). In addition, good economic conditions in the area of residence were significantly related to increases in the employment and income of welfare leavers (Sawhill & Haskins, 2002).

Non-Financial Work Incentive Policies

Few studies have explored the effects that non-financial work incentive policies of states, such as lifetime limits and sanctions for noncompliance with work requirements, have on the employment and economic status of former welfare recipients (Loprest & Wissoker, 2002; Grogger, 2001; Pavetti & Bloom, 2001). The provision of lifetime limits was believed to motivate welfare recipients to participate in work long before they exhaust their 60 months, because the provision might motivate recipients to save their time for a possible time of greater need in the future (Pavetti & Bloom, 2001; Bloom et al., 1998). However, Grogger (2001) found that although lifetime limits had a significant effect on increasing the employment of single mothers on welfare, they had no significant impact on increasing the family income of welfare recipients.

Sanctions were intended to facilitate the work participation of welfare recipients who are receiving full welfare benefits (Coe et al., 1998). Sanctions were positively related to the work incentives and employment of welfare recipients (Loprest & Wissoker, 2002). Rector and Youssef (1999) found that full-check sanctions were significantly related to reductions in welfare caseloads. Hofferth, Stanhope, and Harris (2000) found that stringent sanctions were related to more rapid exits from welfare with employment, while partial sanctions were not enough to affect most welfare recipients.

Financial Work Incentive Policies

The Medicaid program has played an important role in reducing the high risk of low-income families who do not receive needed health care (Lieberman & Mancuso, 2001). However, after the 1996 welfare reform, some families who left welfare were mistakenly terminated from the Medicaid program or were not provided an effective opportunity to apply for Medicaid (Quint & Widom, 2001). The fear of losing Medicaid discouraged some welfare recipients from staying off welfare (Coe et al., 1998). The food stamp program supported poor working families with gross incomes up to 130 percent of the poverty line (Greenstein & Guyer, 2001). However, the 1996 welfare reform law made it more difficult for eligible people to access the food stamp program. In 1997, among families with children 66 percent of those on the food stamp program ceased to receive food stamps.

Previous research has indicated that childcare and transportation assistance were significantly related to the ability to leave welfare, to obtain and hold a job, and to increase family income (Zimmerman et al., 1999). Furthermore, the Federal Earned Income Tax Credit (EITC), a refundable tax credit for low-income families, has significantly increased the income of female-headed families who move from welfare to full-time work (Meyer & Rosenbaum, 1999; Cancian & Meyer, 2000).

Based on previous studies, this study explores how non-financial and financial work incentive policies have influenced the socioeconomic status of welfare leavers in an economically disadvantaged area. Moreover, it examines whether factors such as human capital, family or individual factors (e.g., marital status), and environmental factors influence the socioeconomic status of welfare leavers.

METHODS

Data and Sample

The study uses the 1999 data of the West Virginia University's Welfare Reform Research Team, which surveyed welfare cases that were closed during 1998. The survey was designed in consultation with experts from within and outside West Virginia such as faculties, WV officials, welfare case workers, welfare recipients, and welfare reform advocates. During the summer of 1999, surveys were mailed to a random sample of 2,500 former adult recipients of WV WORKS (child-only cases were excluded). To increase the response rate of mailed surveys, respondents were offered $15. Five hundred eighty surveys (23.2 percent) were returned by the post office as undeliverable, resulting in a sample size of 1,920 former recipients. A total of 962 surveys were completed and returned, for a response rate of 50.1 percent. With a 95 percent confidence interval and a margin of error of plus or minus four percent, samples of this size provide an accurate representation of the experiences of all 18,259 cases of those who left welfare in 1998 (Manheim & Rich, 1986). Moreover, a review of fee requests shows that the respondents matched reasonably the total sample from which they were drawn (Locke & Potter, 2004).

Table 1 shows the sample's demographic characteristics, which were compared with the demographic characteristics of all WV WORKS adult recipients in 1998. This study's sample is similar to the population of all WV WORKS adults in 1998 in many aspects. All 55 counties are represented in the sample. The age distribution of the respondents (82.2% in their 20s and 30s) is similar to the age distribution of the recipients (79.8% in their 20s and 30s). The gender of the respondents (women: 82.2% and men: 17.8%) is similar to the gender of adult WV WORKS recipients in 1998 (women: 79.2% and men: 20.2%). Moreover, the ethnicity of the respondents (White: 91.7%, Black: 5.8%, and others: 2.5%) is similar to the ethnicity of 1998 recipients (White: 93.3%, Black: 6.1%, and others: 0.6%). There was an expected difference between the marital status of respondents (married: 38.8%, never married: 26%, and others: 35.2%) and WV WORKS recipients in 1998 (married: 31.7%, never married: 37.5%, and others: 30.8%), expected because one of the reasons for leaving WV WORKS was a change in marital status. Furthermore, there was comparative difference in education between the respondents (no high school degree/GED: 30.4% and high

TABLE 1. Demographic Comparison of 1998 State Data of WV WORKS Recipients to Survey Sample of WV WORKS Leavers (in percent)

		Survey Data[1]	State Data[2]
Age	In 20s and 30s	82.2	79.8
Gender	Male	17.8	20.2
	Female	82.2	79.8
Race	White	91.7	93.3
	Black	5.8	6.1
	Others	2.5	0.6
Marital status	Married	38.8	31.7
	Never married	26.0	37.5
	Others (widowed, divorced, separated, etc.)	35.2	30.8
Education	No high school degree/GED	30.4	44.7
	High school degree or greater	69.6	54.7
Job training	Yes	6.8	—
	No	93.2	—
Disability	Yes	15.2	—
	No	84.8	—
Living area	Cities or suburbs	24.2	—
	Small towns	36.5	—
	Isolated areas	39.3	—

Sources: 1. 1999 West Virginia Survey of the West Virginia University's Welfare Reform Research Team.
2. U.S. Department of Health and Human Services 1999.

school degree/GED or greater: 69.6%) and 1998 recipients (no high school degree/GED: 44.7% and high school degree/GED or greater: 54.7%).

Variables and Measurements

Independent Variables

Respondents were asked to report how many total months of WV WORKS/TANF eligibility they had left. Respondents chose from among five categories: 1 to 12 months (coded as 1); 13 to 24 months (coded as 2); 25 to 36 months (coded as 3); 37 to 48 months (coded as 4); and 49 to 60 months (coded as 5). Individuals who were sanctioned and had lost their eligibility were coded 1, with the others coded as 0. Respondents who were receiving Medicaid, food stamps, childcare assistance, transportation assistance, or the Earned Income Tax Credits (EITC) were coded as 1, while respondents who were not receiving them were coded as 0.

If respondents did not have a high school degree/GED, that fact was coded as 1. If respondents had a high school degree/GED, it was coded as 2. If they had a college or graduate degree, it was coded as 3. Individuals who were married were coded as 1, those who were divorced, widowed, or separated were coded as 2, and those who had never been married were coded as 3. Respondents who were African Americans were coded as 1, those who were Asians, Native Americans, and Hispanics or Latinos were coded as 2, while those who were Whites are coded as 3. Individuals who had taken job training, a disability, or lived in isolated areas were coded as 1, while others were coded as 0.

Dependent Variables

Respondents who had left and stayed off WV WORKS for the previous year were coded as 1, while others were coded as 0. Respondents who were currently employed were coded as 1, while those not employed were coded as 0. Respondents were asked to indicate if they expected their total household income for 1999 to be less than $5,000 (coded as 1), $5,001-10,000 (coded as 2), $10,001-15,000 (coded as 3), $15,001-20,000 (coded as 4), $20,001-25,000 (coded as 5), or greater than $25,000 (coded as 6). In addition, all respondents were asked to compare their financial status while on WV WORKS to their status after WV WORKS. Respondents were coded as follows: much better off (coded as 5); better off (coded as 4); about the same (coded as 3); worse off (coded as 2); or much worse off (coded as 1).

Data Analyses

This study uses two statistical methods to analyze the data. First, it uses a logistic regression method because two dependent variables ("Welfare exit" and "Employed now") are dummy variables (Mertler & Vannatta, 2001). The effects of the independent variables on the dependent variables are expressed in the odds ratios. Second, the study uses an ordinal regression method because the dependent variables ("Household income" and "Financial status") are ordinal variables (Long, 1997). These methods show how work incentive variables and other independent variables influence the socioeconomic status of welfare leavers.

RESULTS

Characteristics of the Main Variables

Twenty-nine percent of the respondents had 1 to 12 months of TANF eligibility remaining, 21.3 percent had 13 to 24 months, 11.5 percent had 25 to 36 months, 15.8 percent had 37 to 48 months, and 22.4 percent had 49 to 60 months. Slightly more than four percent (4.1%) reported being sanctioned and losing their eligibility for welfare benefits. About 60 percent of the sample was receiving Medicaid and more than half of the respondents were receiving food stamps. Only 8.3 percent of respondents were receiving childcare assistance and only 3.7 percent were receiving transportation assistance. Around 21 percent of the respondents reported receiving the Earned Income Tax Credit (EITC).

In the current study, 62.6 percent of the sample left and stayed off TANF. Fewer than half of welfare leavers successfully entered the labor force after leaving welfare. About 70 percent of welfare leavers expected their total household income for 1999 to be less than $10,000. A total of 25.9 percent of the respondents indicated that they were either worse off or much worse off financially since leaving WV WORKS, 42.6 percent indicated being either much better off or better off financially, and 31.4 percent indicated being about the same as when they were enrolled in WV WORKS.

Multivariate Analyses

Table 2 contains the results from the logistic regression for the "Welfare exit" and "Employed now" model. There were no multicollinearity problems because the VIF did not exceed 10.0. The results show that people who were receiving food stamps and EITC were less likely than those who were not receiving food stamps and EITC to leave and stay off welfare. However, people who were married were about five times more likely than never married people to stay off welfare. African Americans were over eleven times more likely than Whites to stay off welfare.

TABLE 2. Estimated Coefficients of Logistic Regression Predicting *Welfare Exit* and *Employed Now* of Welfare Leavers

	Welfare Exit (n = 962)			Employed Now (n = 912)		
	B[1]	SE[2]	Exp(B)[3]	B[1]	SE[2]	Exp(B)[3]
Lifetime limits	−2.71	.149	.762	.354*	.171	1.425
Sanctions	−1.081	1.138	.339	−4.617*	1.984	.010
Medicaid	−0.75	.515	.928	−1.064*	.537	.345
Food stamps	−2.506**	.841	.082	−.881	.702	.415
Childcare assistance	.853	.693	2.347	2.459**	.933	11.691
Transportation assistance	−.339	1.035	.712	.293	1.185	1.341
EITC	−1.208*	.536	.299	.173	.617	3.231
Education (vs. no high school degree/GED)						
High school degree/GED	−.151	.606	.860	.030	.647	2.801
College or graduate degree	.128	.744	1.137	2.457**	.899	11.673
Job training	−.454	.743	.635	.436	.795	1.547
Disability	−.200	.710	.819	−1.465	.912	.231
Marital status (vs. never married)						
Married	1.564**	.554	4.778	−.562	.628	.570
Others	−.106	.559	.900	−.872	.668	.418
Race (vs. Whites)						
African Americans	2.434*	.974	11.409	.100	.859	1.105
Others	6.644	22.251	768.104	2.616	22.263	13.684
Isolated area	.240	.479	1.271	−.671	.543	.511
Constant	2.935**	1.089		−.376	1.038	
Model Chi-square (16d.f.)	37.724**			52.612***		
Pseudo R square (Cox and Snell)	.261			.357		

*p ≤ .05, ** p ≤ .01, *** p ≤ .001
[1]Standardized coefficient, [2]Standard errors, [3]Odds ratios

The results indicate that people who had more months of eligibility remaining for TANF were around one and a half times more likely than those with fewer months of eligibility remaining to have jobs. People who had been sanctioned and lost eligibility for welfare benefits were less likely than those who had not been sanctioned to have jobs. People who were receiving Medicaid were less likely than those without Medicaid to have jobs. On the other hand, people who were receiving childcare assistance were over eleven times more likely than those without childcare assistance to have jobs. People who had college or graduate degrees were over eleven times more likely than those without high school degrees to have jobs.

Table 3 contains the ordinal regression results for the "Household income" and "Financial status" model. There were no multicollinearity problems because VIF did not exceed 10.0. The results indicate that people who were receiving EITC were more likely than those who were not receiving EITC to expect high household income.

The results indicate that people who were receiving EITC were more likely than those who were not receiving EITC to be financially better off after leaving welfare. Widowed, divorced, or separated people were more likely than never married people to be financially better off. Asians, Native Americans, or Hispanics were less likely than Whites to be financially better off. People who lived in isolated places were less likely than those who lived in small towns or suburbs to be financially better off after leaving welfare.

DISCUSSION/POLICY IMPLICATIONS

This study found that people who had more months of eligibility remaining for TANF were more likely than those with fewer months of eligibility to have jobs. This finding is different from the findings of previous research that lifetime limits facilitated welfare leavers having jobs before anyone reached their lifetime limits (Bloom et al., 1998). This finding indicates that in an economically disadvantaged area, lifetime limits do not induce welfare leavers to work. Lifetime limits hasten job searches and lead to poorer job matches (Grogger, 2001). As a result, lifetime limits do not promote welfare leavers having stable jobs with increasing wages (Vartanian & McNamara, 2000). Policy makers need to consider the extension of lifetime limits, as well as to pay attention to welfare leavers who have exhausted their 5-year lifetime limits because frequently they are not able to obtain jobs. For example, Dilger

TABLE 3. Estimated Coefficients of Ordinal Regression Predicting *Household Income* and *Financial Status* of Welfare Leavers

	Household Income (n = 836)		Financial Status (n = 786)	
	B[1]	SE[2]	B[1]	SE[2]
Lifetime limits	−6.004	.121	.193	.119
Sanctions	.965	.874	−.989	.831
Medicaid	−.819	.427	.359	.413
Food stamps	6.805	.507	−.936	.495
Childcare assistance	−.210	.556	.470	.559
Transportation assistance	−.904	.927	−.427	.831
EITC	.853*	.426	1.319**	.452
Education (vs. no high school degree/GED)				
High school degree/GED	.511	.499	.766	.469
College or graduate degree	.923	.590	.826	.602
Job training	−.629	.606	.359	.623
Disability	.255	.611	−.516	.571
Marital status (vs. never married)				
Married	.314	.448	.615	.431
Others	.221	.446	1.154*	.453
Race (vs. Whites)				
African Americans	1.345	.606	−1.080	.623
Others	−1.728	1.926	−3.882*	1.933
Isolated area	−.201	.395	−.842**	.387
Model Chi-square (16d.f.)	22.111		35.741**	
Pseudo R square (Cox and Snell)	.175		.256	

*p ≤ .05, **p ≤ .01, ***p ≤ .001
[1]Standardized coefficient, [2]Standard errors

et al. (2004) found that in an economically disadvantaged state, only about one-quarter of the respondents who had exhausted their 5 years of TANF eligibility were employed, while over 90 percent of the respondents had less than $10,000 household income.

The current study found that people who had been sanctioned for noncompliance with work requirements were less likely than those who had not been sanctioned to have jobs. Some studies have showed that sanctions motivate welfare recipients to leave welfare with employment (Coe et al., 1998; Loprest & Wissoker, 2002). Pavetti and Bloom (2001) insisted that because of their mental and physical health problems, many welfare recipients were unable to comply with work requirements, and so received sanctions. Moreover, sanctions caused people who were unskilled and uneducated to leave welfare without jobs. As a result, sanctions negatively influenced the self-sufficiency of welfare leavers in an economically disadvantaged area because disabled and uneducated people rarely find jobs where there is long-term recession.

This study's findings contain important policy implications for welfare reform reauthorization (Fremstad & Parrot, 2004). Reauthorization should focus on increasing financial work incentive policies and emphasizing human capital development strategies rather than imposing non-financial work incentive policies. Childcare assistance significantly influences welfare leavers to have jobs (Zimmerman et al., 1999). Many researchers have argued that childcare assistance was a key factor in welfare leavers working continuously or having stable jobs (Tweedie et al., 1999). However, only 8.3 percent of respondents in this study were receiving childcare assistance from the state government, less than the 11.4 percent in nationwide data (Urban Institute, 1999). In rural areas, single mothers have great difficulty in accessing childcare centers because childcare resources were rare and far away from residence or place of employment. In West Virginia, over 95 percent of respondents reported that they could not find childcare when they needed to go to work.

In economically disadvantaged areas, there is often an inadequate childcare support system (Marson et al., 2000). Even though states provide childcare for welfare leavers, it often does not appropriately meet their needs. For example, in the cases of single mothers, if their children become sick, the mothers have to take care of them instead of working. This often results in the leavers being fired by employers and forces them to return to welfare. In addition, Marson et al. (2000) argued that public transportation did not appropriately provide welfare leavers access to specific work places. In their study, vans did not have a regular route and schedule, so welfare leavers could not arrive on time to work. This current study suggests that policy makers in economically disadvantaged states should provide appropriate services for welfare leavers to work continuously within their environmental structures.

In the current study, the EITC is significantly associated with expecting high household income and being financially better off after leaving welfare, a finding that is consistent with previous studies (Meyer & Rosenbaum, 1999). Grogger (2001) and Coe et al. (1998) have argued that the EITC was a significant factor in increasing the employment and family income of welfare leavers. Policy makers need to gradually increase the role of the EITC to facilitate the employment and income of welfare recipients and leavers.

This study found that there were negative relationships between financial work incentive policies such as food stamps and Medicaid and the employment and economic status of welfare leavers because people who had jobs and high family income were not likely to have food stamps and Medicaid (Coe et al., 1998). However, many welfare leavers who are eligible do not participate in these programs. Loss of food stamps and Medicaid is a strong disincentive for welfare leavers to continue working (Ellwood & Ku, 1998). This study supports permanent reauthorization of the Transitional Medical Assistance (TMA) and the extension of its eligibility for low-income families (Fremstad & Parrot, 2004). Furthermore, decision makers need to clarify administrative processes and rules so that eligible welfare leavers will have access to these programs.

This study found that high education among welfare leavers is a significant and positive variable affecting employment, which is consistent with previous research (Tweedie et al., 1999; Holzer, 2002). Working is an important factor in the independence of welfare recipients (Cancian & Meyer, 2000). However, many welfare leavers in economically disadvantaged areas did not have appropriate work skills and resources to continue working. The findings of this study provide support for educational programs for low-income families, such as Adult Basic Education Classes, Job Services, Job Search, etc. However, in the current study, only a small number of welfare leavers had taken educational programs when they enrolled in WV WORKS because state government focused on work first policies. The attention of policy makers is needed to increase stable jobs and income for welfare leavers with emphasis on educational programs relating to work or job training. In addition, Martinson and Strawn (2003) have argued that mixed service approaches, which combine strong linkages to employers and employment services with education and job skills training were more effective than welfare-to-work programs, which focused solely on job search and related activities.

Paying special attention to the needs of former welfare recipients with bad health conditions that limit work is needed, even though this study did not find significant effects of health conditions on the socioeconomic status of those leaving welfare. Danziger and Seefeldt (2002) have argued that physical disabilities might be preventing economic opportunities among former welfare recipients. The results of data analysis show that 84.4 percent of those who had mental or physical disability made less than $10,000 per year compared with 75.4 percent of people without disability. This study suggests that former welfare recipients who have physical disabilities should have better access to public health care and health insurance. In light of these conclusions, policy makers need to expand the 20 percent of the federal caseload exemption rate for states with higher percentages of welfare recipients with disabilities (Latimer, 2004).

In the current study, married welfare leavers were more likely than unmarried people to get off welfare, a finding that is consistent with previous work (Sandefur & Cook, 1998). The respondents who had been or were married were more likely than never married people to be financially better off after leaving welfare. These findings show that since spouses financially support married welfare leavers, the welfare leavers were more likely than their never married counterparts to leave welfare programs without jobs. Latimer (2004) found that even though married mothers who left welfare were significantly less likely than never married people to be employed, they had more financial resources coming into the household. These findings seem to indicate the importance of marriage in staying off welfare and in increasing the economic status of welfare leavers. The results support $1.5 billion earmarked for marriage promotion in the House TANF reauthorization bill (Fremstad & Parrot, 2004).

In the current study, Whites were less likely than Blacks to stay off welfare, but Whites were more likely than Asians, Native Americans, or Hispanics to be financially better off, which is consistent with previous research (Holzer, 2000). African American welfare recipients were more likely than Whites to leave welfare because of administrative problems and complex program rules (Gooden, 1998). Finegold and Staveteig (2002: 215) insist that "[b]ias in the use of [caseworkers'] discretion, whether intentional or unintentional, can result in racial and ethnic disparities in the receipt of benefits." The results of West Virginia survey data show that 47.7 percent of African American welfare cases were closed by the DHHR, while only 38.1 percent of White welfare cases were closed. Nearly seven percent (6.7%) of African American welfare cases were sanctioned, but only 4.1 percent of White cases were sanctioned. Moreover, minority low-income families were more likely than Whites to experience food and housing hardship despite extremely positive overall economic conditions (Dupree & Primus, 2001). However, white welfare recipients were more likely to receive help with expenses when they left welfare. Fix and Passel (2002) argued that welfare reform, although not explicitly based on race or ethnicity, has produced unintentional discrimination in work support or work incentive policies toward low-income blacks and immigrant families. Policy makers and case workers need to pay particular attention to minority welfare recipients because they have more barriers to their self-sufficiency than do Whites.

Finally, in an economically disadvantaged state, living in isolated places is a negative factor in welfare leavers being financially better off after leaving welfare, which is consistent with previous research (Sawhill & Haskins, 2002). Policy makers need to consider the effect of place and allow different work incentive policies–both within and across states.

Overall, this study makes significant contributions to existing knowledge about welfare reform by examining the effects of work incentive policies on the socioeconomic status of welfare leavers in an economically disadvantaged area. This study has been uniquely designed to show the isolated impact of non-financial work incentive policies, such as lifetime limits and sanctions and financial work incentive policies, on the socioeconomic status of welfare leavers. Even though this study uses 1999 survey data, the findings may help policy makers adapt current work incentive policies. This is because few research studies have focused on analyzing the effects of lifetime limits and sanctions on the socioeconomic status of welfare leavers in rural areas. In addition, this study contributes to find important determinants of the socioeconomic status of welfare leavers.

However, the limitations of the present study should be considered when interpreting these findings. As this study examined the impact of work incentive policies on welfare leavers after only three years, there are limitations in analyzing the impact of work incentive policies after the five-year welfare reform authorization. It is difficult to generalize these findings to all states because this study used survey data from one economically disadvantaged state in analyzing the impact of work incentive policies on the socioeconomic status of welfare leavers. Also, the study did not compare rural and urban areas in states in analyzing the effects of work incentive policies on the socioeconomic status of welfare leavers.

Thus, future studies are needed to examine the effect of work incentive policies on the socioeconomic well-being of welfare leavers, using national data after the TANF period of five years. Longitudinal studies should be conducted to understand the functions of work incentive policies of states on the socioeconomic well-being of welfare leavers. Finally, comparison studies are needed to understand the effects of work incentive policies in different economic conditions of states on the socioeconomic status of welfare leavers.

REFERENCES

Bloom, D., Farrel, M., & Fink, B. (2002). *Welfare time limits: State policies, implementation, and effects on families*. New York: Manpower Demonstration Research Corporation.

Cancian, M., & Meyer, D. R. (2000). Work after welfare: Women's work effort, occupation, and economic well-being. *Social Work Research, 24*(2), 69-86.

Coe, N. B., Acs, G., Lerman, R. I., & Watson, K. (1998). *Does work pay?: A summary of the work incentives under TANF*. Series A, No. A-28. Washington, DC: Urban Institute.

Danziger, S. K., & Seefeldt, K. S. (2002). Barriers to employment and the 'Hard to Serve': Implications for services, sanctions, and time limits. *Focus, 22*(1), 76-81.

Dilger, R. J. (2004). Cash assistance and social welfare policy in the United States: The political and institutional context. In R. J. Dilger (Ed.), *Welfare reform in West Virginia: Lessons from the mountain* state (pp. 55-106). WV: West Virginia University Press.

Dilger, R. J., Blakely, E., Latimer, M., Locke, B., Plein, L. C., Potter, L., & Williams, D. (2004). WV WORKS 2003: Perspectives of former recipients who have exhausted their 60 months of program eligibility. *The West Virginia Public Affairs Reporter, 21*(2), 2-20.

Dupree, A., & Primus, W. (2001). Declining share of children lived with single mothers in the late 1990s. Washington, DC: Center on Budget and Policy Priorities.

Ellwood, M., & Ku, L. (1998). Welfare and immigration problems: Unintended side effects for Medicaid. *Health Affairs, 17*(3), 137-151.

Finegold, K., & Staveteig, S. (2002). Race, ethnicity, and welfare reform. In A. Weil & K. Finegold (Eds.), *Welfare reform: The next act* (pp. 203-224). Washington, DC: Urban Institute Press.

Fix, M., & Passel, J. S. (2002). Assessing welfare reform's immigrant provisions. In A. Weil & K. Finegold (Eds.), *Welfare reform: The next act* (pp. 179-202). Washington, DC: Urban Institute Press.

Fremstad, S., & Parrot, S. (2004). The Senate Finance Committee's TANF reauthorization bill. Washington, DC: Center on Budget and Policy Priorities.

Gooden, S. T. (1998). All things not being equal: Differences in caseworker support toward Black and White welfare clients. *Harvard Journal of African American Public Policy, 4*(1), 23-33.

Greenstein, R., & Guyer, J. (2001). Supporting work through Medicaid and food stamps. In R. Blank & R. Haskins (Eds.), *The new world of welfare* (pp. 335-368). Washington, DC: Brookings Institution Press.

Grogger, J. (2001). The effects of time limits and other policy changes on welfare use, work, and income among female-headed family. NBER Working Paper 8153, National Bureau of Economic Research.

Hofferth, S. L., Stanhope, S., & Harris, K. M. (2000). Exiting welfare in the 1990s: Did public policy influence recipients' behavior. Research Report No. 01-469, Population Studies Center at the Institute for Social Research, University of Michigan.

Holzer, H. J. (2000). Career advancement prospects and strategies for low-wage minority workers. Washington, DC: Urban Institute.

Karger, H. J., & Stoesz, D. (2002). *American social welfare policy* (4th ed.). New York: Longman.

Latimer, M. (2004). Between a rock and a hard place–The socioeconomic status of former TANF recipients in West Virginia. *Sociological Spectrum, 24*(1), 93-123.

Lieberman, C., & Mancuso, D. C. (2001). Are California's welfare leavers staying off public assistance?: Welfare recidivism and use of non-cash aid since welfare reform. *California Policy Review, 1*(2), 1-11.

Locke, B. L., & Potter, L. A. (2004). Voices from the mountains. In T. L. Scales & C. L. Streeter (Eds.), *Rural social work: Building and sustaining community assets* (pp. 263-274). CA: Thomson & Brooks/Cole.

Long, J. S. (1997). *Regression models for categorical and limited dependent variables*. CA: Sage Publication, Inc.

Loprest, P., & Wissoker, D. (2002). Employment and welfare reform in the National Survey of America's Families. The New Federalism Discussion Paper No. 02-04. Washington, DC: Urban Institute.

Marson, S. M., & Powell, R. M. (2000). Churners: A focus group analysis of the return rate of former rural TANF recipients [Welfare recidivism in Robeson county, N.C.]. *Policy and Practice of Public Human Services, 58*(4), 44-49.

Martinson, K., & Strawn, J. (2003). Built to last: Why skills matter for long-run success in welfare reform. Washington, DC: Center for Law and Social Policy.

Mertler, C. A., & Vannatta, R. A. (2001). *Advanced and multivariate statistical methods: Practical application and interpretation*. CA: Pyrczak Publishing.

Meyer, B. D., & Rosenbaum, D. T. (1999). Making single mothers work: Recent tax and welfare policy and its effects. *National Tax Journal, 53*(4), 1027-1062.

Pavetti, L., & Bloom, D. (2001). State sanctions and time limits. In R. Blank & R. Haskins (Eds.), *The new world of welfare* (pp. 245-269). Washington, DC: Brookings Institution Press.

Plein, L. C. (2001). Welfare reform in a hard place: The West Virginia experience. *Rockefeller Report, No. 13*. New York: The Nelson A. Rockefeller Institute of Government.

Quint, J., & Widom, R. (2001). Post-TANF and food stamp and Medicaid benefits: Factors that aid or impede their receipt. New York: Manpower Demonstration Research Corporation.

Rector, R. E., & Youssef, S. E. (1999). The determinants of welfare caseload decline. A Report of the Heritage Center for Data Analysis. The Heritage Foundation.

Sandefur, G. D., & Cook, S. T. (1998). Permanent exits from public assistance: The impact of duration, family, and work. *Social Forces, 77*(2), 763-787.

Sawhill, I., & Haskins, R. (2002). Welfare reform and the work support system. Policy Brief No. 17, March. Washington, DC: Brookings Institution.

Tweedie, J., Reichert, D., & O'Connor, M. (1999). Tracking recipients after they leave welfare: Summaries of new state tracking studies. National Conference of State Legislatures.

Urban Institute. (1999). *National survey of America's families*. Washington, DC: Urban Institute.

U.S. Census Bureau. (2003). *Current population survey*. Retrieved from the Web January 10, 2004. http://www.bls.census.gov/cps/cpsmain.htm.

U.S. Department of Health and Human Services (DHHS). (2000). *Temporary Assistance for Needy Families Program (TANF): Third annual report to Congress.* Washington, DC: U.S. Department of Health and Human Services.

U.S. General Accounting Office. (1999). Welfare reform: Information on former recipients' status. GAO/HEHS-99-48. April. Washington, DC: U.S. Government Printing Office.

Vartanian, T. P., & McNamara, J. M. (2000). Work and economic outcomes after welfare. *Journal of Sociology & Social Welfare, 27*(2), 41-77.

Zimmerman, J., Dewees, S., Reinschmiedt, L., & Hirschl, T. (1999). *Rural America and welfare reform: An overview assessment.* Rural Policy Research Institute, University of Missouri, Columbia, MO.

Shadow Welfare II: Tax Expenditures and Corporate Welfare in the States

Christopher S. Blanchard
Daniel D. Huff

SUMMARY. Tax expenditures are any exemption, credit, deduction, or exclusion from the payment of taxes. At the state level, such expenditures often remain unaccounted for, create little economic development, and leave state and local governments with reduced resources for funding basic services such as fire, police, schools, and other general welfare spending. This paper illustrates methods state and local governments use to grant large tax breaks, the resulting financial problems legislators typically solve by raising individual taxes or cutting spending, and the implications for social welfare practitioners. *[Article copies available for a fee from The Haworth Document Delivery Service: 1-800-HAWORTH. E-mail address: <docdelivery@haworthpress.com> Website: <http://www.HaworthPress.com> © 2005 by The Haworth Press, Inc. All rights reserved.]*

KEYWORDS. State policy, local government, tax expenditures, tax policy

---

Christopher S. Blanchard and Daniel D. Huff are affiliated with the School of Social Work, Boise State University, 1910 University Drive, Boise, ID 83725-1940.

[Haworth co-indexing entry note]: "Shadow Welfare II: Tax Expenditures and Corporate Welfare in the States." Blanchard, Christopher S., and Daniel D. Huff. Co-published simultaneously in *The Social Policy Journal* (The Haworth Press, Inc.) Vol. 4, No. 3/4, 2005, pp. 127-142; and: *Cutting-Edge Social Policy Research* (ed: Richard Hoefer) The Haworth Press, Inc., 2005, pp. 127-142. Single or multiple copies of this article are available for a fee from The Haworth Document Delivery Service [1-800-HAWORTH, 9:00 a.m. - 5:00 p.m. (EST). E-mail address: docdelivery@haworthpress.com].

Available online at http://www.haworthpress.com/web/SPJ

doi:10.1300/J185v04n03_08

Tax shelters are to democracy what pollution is to the environment. When companies spew toxic wastes into the air and water, they are saving money by not running cleaner operations and by making everyone else bear that cost through acid rain, fouled water, and diseases like cancer. When they use tax dodges . . . they are saving money by not paying the price of maintaining the civilization that has made their success possible. (Johnston, 2003)

INTRODUCTION

In a previous edition of this journal, Bader, Huff, and Reynolds examined the trend of shifting government resources away from working people to the more affluent through the use of federal tax expenditures (Bader, Huff, & Reynolds, 2003). Tax expenditures are any exemption, credit, deduction, or exclusion from the payment of taxes (Brunori, 2001). This earlier study found that the federal government allowed corporations and individuals to pay less than their fair share of taxes, thereby weakening potential federal responses to emerging social problems, as well as maintaining social welfare spending at current levels. The authors demonstrated that tax expenditures are by their very nature regressive, and amount to hundreds of billions of dollars in uncollected revenues (Bader, Huff, & Reynolds, 2003).

This paper examines a practice even more elusive than federal tax expenditures–state tax expenditures. Today, twenty-nine states in the nation calculate an expenditure budget, but only fourteen make that report available electronically (Mikesell, 2002). Arizona's 2001-2002 expenditure budget runs 177 pages, and includes no aggregate total for all expenditures (Arizona Department of Revenue, 2002). Twenty-one states have no accounting for the enormity of the revenues forgone to tax expenditures (Mikesell, 2002). Thus even when the information on tax expenditures is available, it may be difficult to obtain, or requires more computation before the information is useful.

Tracking expenditures is made even more difficult because state government budget operatives calculate tax expenditure budgets in several different ways (Mikesell, 2002). One method is the *revenue reducer* method, which lists all changes in law reducing revenues to the state. A second method is based on *reference tax law*. Using this methodology, analysts normatively determine what is and what is not a standard part of the tax code. Thus, they may or may not include all portions of law that reduce revenues. For example, as we later discuss in this paper, the *single sales factor* formula for calculating corporate income tax, adopted by many states, substantially reduces revenues, but lawmakers are free to claim this as a standard part of the tax code and not count it as a revenue reducing mechanism. In some instances they ignore its effect entirely.

Under the reference tax law methodology, ". . . some exemptions and exclusions are part of the normal baseline, not preferences" (Mikesell, 2002). Using this methodology, states are under no obligation to consider "benchmark(s) driven by a fundamental tax policy logic" (Mikesell, 2002). In other words, lawmakers may consider any alteration in the tax code, "standard." Twenty states use this methodology. The state of Washington, which uses the reference tax law methodology, is under no obligation to account for much of the $3.2 billion (Evergreen Freedom Foundation, 2004) in tax exemptions it recently granted Boeing to entice the aerospace manufacturer to add 2,000-3,000 new jobs in the state (Wallace, 2003). Thus, the State subsidized Boeing's payroll to the tune of $53,000 per job, per year, for the next 20 years–and may or may not account for this expenditure in any budget. With all the various methodologies and definitions of what is and what is not an expenditure, quantifying all state tax expenditures proves difficult.

From a social welfare perspective state tax expenditures are arguably more deleterious to the general welfare than federal tax expenditures. There are several reasons for this. First, federal policy beginning with the Reagan Administration's shift to block grants, and continuing with the Clinton Administration's welfare reform in 1996, shifted more and more of the social welfare burden to the states. Second, unlike the federal government, states operate within the confines of constitutionally prescribed balanced budget requirements. Third, state tax systems in general are more regressive than federal taxes due to reliance upon sales taxes. With the soft economy over the last several years, legislators are considering more tax breaks to business in efforts to jump start state economies. All these trends present a serious threat to general welfare spending. Thus, the outcome of the guns and butter debate has never been clearer: states can either spend money on tax breaks for business, or spend money on the general welfare–and all signs point to the former.

State governments increasingly generate revenues by taxing individuals through personal income taxes, and sales and excise taxes; there has been a calculated shift away from corporate taxation. In 1950, personal income taxes constituted 9.3% of state revenues. By 1970, that portion grew to 19%; by 1998, 34% (Brunori, 2001). State lawmakers are shifting the burden to individual taxpayers. The arcane measures this paper describes produce that shift to other revenue generators, for example, sales and use taxes, excise taxes, fees, and personal income taxes. In 2004, 94% of the $9.6 billion in tax increases levied by state governments fell on individuals, mostly in the form of highly regressive sales and excise taxes (National Association of State Budget Officers [NASBO], 2003).

Since the bursting of the high-tech bubble, nearly every state faces budget deficits (NASBO, 2003). These deficits, however, are not only due to an overall weak economy but also because of structural problems in state tax codes, for example, reliance upon regressive tax instruments such as sales and excise taxes; absence of taxes on services and remote sales which constitute the bulk of today's economic activity, and; continued use of corporate tax expenditures. In fiscal years 2005 and 2006, many states will balance their budgets by cutting social welfare spending rather than addressing the elephant in the room: tax codes with a preponderance of loopholes and decades of dispensing fiscal favors to powerful interest groups.

SOUTH CAROLINA: A CASE STUDY

The fiscal problems in South Carolina offer an example. In the mid 1990s, partly as a result of tax expenditures aimed at attracting new business, South Carolina drew nearly 1,400 new businesses creating 200,000 new jobs. This economic growth brought 300,000 new residents–and a correspondingly high demand for government services (Hancock, 1999). The demand for new infrastructure and government services, in fact, far outstripped government revenues. Meanwhile, South Carolina's per capita crime rate climbed 19% between 1987 and 1997; four in ten homes remained unconnected to sewers; South Carolina posted the lowest SAT scores in the nation and had one of the nation's highest infant mortality rates; 35 schools reported leaky roofs and two-dozen complained of worn out carpet (Hancock, 1999). At the heart of the state's problems: aggressive use of tax expenditures in an effort to jumpstart the state's economy. As Jay Hancock of the South Carolina Sun reported:

> BMW has never paid South Carolina's 5 percent tax on corporate profits and shows no signs of doing so for years. . . . The company pays $1 a year to lease its $36 million piece of land. It pays no land tax to Spartanburg County . . . corporate income tax revenue has

> fallen by 6 percent since 1994 . . . other business-tax collections are languishing, too. Across the state, local property revenue on business equipment plummeted 13 percent from 1993-1997. (Hancock, 1999)

With expenditures rising and revenues falling, South Carolina legislators quickly unveiled revenue enhancement proposals. In Charleston County, county administrators increased property taxes, and water fees, implemented a one-percent sales tax, and a three-percent phone tax (Hancock, 1999). Surrounding counties quintupled home inspection fees, increased trash fees, and implemented telephone taxes of their own (Hancock, 1999). This flurry of legislative activity clearly demonstrates the legislator's propensity for levying regressive tax measures during times of fiscal crisis–individuals were paying the taxes that corporations were not. Eventually, South Carolina amassed $57 billion of infrastructure needs (Hancock, 1999), and a budget deficit of $700 million (Center for Budget and Policy Priorities [CBPP], 2003c). Municipalities in South Carolina brokered 200 tax abatement deals with individual corporations before keeping track of the transactions (Hancock, 1999).

Further, between 1994 and 1999, South Carolina's average manufacturing wage grew only 5 percent, while the national wage growth rate averaged 12 percent (Hancock, 1999). Even after the mass of tax expenditures, by 1999 manufacturing jobs in South Carolina paid on average $33,949–well below the national average of $41,918 (Bureau of Labor Statistics [BLS], 1999). By 2002, manufacturing wages in the state averaged $37,604, but the state had lost 381 manufacturing firms (BLS, 2002). Though the jobs departed, many things remained: the budget deficit, an inadequate infrastructure, and a growing population with many needs.

CUTTING PROGRAMS, LEAVING LOOPHOLES

South Carolina presents one of the more glaring examples of sacrificing social welfare and other government spending in order to provide business tax breaks. It is a trend that is quite common. The National Association of State Budget Officers calculated that 2002 and 2003 were record years for program cuts at the state level. In 2002, 38 states combined to cut their program budgets by $13.7 billion. In 2003, 40 states made budget cuts totaling $11.8 billion (NASBO, 2003). In its 2003

Fiscal Survey of the States, NASBO outlined what programs states were cutting:

> During the beginning of the most recent economic downturn, priority programs such as Medicaid, K-12 education, higher education, debt service, public safety, and aid to towns and cities, or those set by predetermined formulas such as school aid, typically have been held harmless from budget cuts. As the state fiscal crunch has lingered during the past two years, these programs now are being cut. (NASBO, 2003)

What surprises many analysts though is not what programs the states decided to cut, but what programs they spared. California's legislators all agreed the only thing they absolutely could not cut was the legislative budget itself. At the same time, they considered a massive corporate tax cut, the institution of a single sales factor formula for corporate income tax calculation (detailed later), and trimmed over $2 billion from the previous year's budget (NASBO, 2003). Montana reduced Temporary Assistance to Needy Families (TANF) payments by 26 percent, and hiked individual taxes $43 million–then cut corporate taxes $48 million (NASBO, 2003; CBPP, 2002). Courts in the state of New York forced legislators to increase TANF housing payments to working poor families (NASBO, 2003), while at the same time and in order to balance the budget, New York legislators passed $3 billion worth of tax increases, including a repeal of the sales tax exemption on clothing and footwear (NASBO, 2003). The clothing and footwear exemption cost the state $449 million annually–not a small sum (NASBO, 2003). It represents, however, only half the amount the state loses each year to loopholes in international tax law (Multistate Tax Commission [MTC], 2003).

Health care spending declined across the board. Thirty-four states reduced or restricted Medicaid eligibility; 35 states reduced benefits; 32 states increased co-payments (NASBO, 2003). Total sales tax increases among the states increasing sales taxes for FY 2004 amounted to $2.6 billion; personal income tax increases totaled $2.4 billion; tobacco and alcohol taxes increased $751 million and "other" taxes and fees levied against individuals for FY 2004 totaled $3 billion (NASBO, 2003). Meanwhile, corporate income taxes increased only $601 million, or less than the combined tax increases on tobacco and alcohol (NASBO,

2003). Only five states closed any kind of corporate tax loophole (NASBO, 2003).

Twenty-two states allow sheltering of corporate income through passive investment corporations (PIC); 20 states allow corporations to create *nowhere income*, income that is subjected to no tax; 26 states define business income in such a manner that allows corporations to escape millions of dollars of taxation annually; 40 states have altered the egalitarian corporate income tax formula created by the Multi-State Tax Commission in 1957, alterations which allow corporations to escape large portions of their tax bill (CBPP, 2003a). These expenditures receive little attention from social welfare advocates. The following sections of the paper describe the impact of some of the more common hidden expenditures–expenditures considered a standard part of tax law, and their costs to state budgets. These expenditures constitute a major, yet often neglected area of the corporate shadow welfare state.

HIDING EXPENDITURES IN THE CORPORATE INCOME TAX LAW

In 1957, the Multi State Tax Commission adopted the "Uniform Division of Income for Tax Purposes Act" (MTC, 2003). This act created a formula for corporate income taxation based upon three things: sales, property, and payroll. Soon, states, lobbyists, and corporations realized this formulation provided a means for influencing economic development. By altering the proportions of the formula, states issued tax breaks rewarding certain types of business. For example, *double weighting* the sales factor reduces the tax liability of corporations with large amounts of property and payrolls in state. Another strategy is the *single sales factor* formula wherein income tax is based solely upon in-state sales; payroll and property become irrelevant. These formula alterations benefit large manufacturers who typically export a high proportion of their products, shifting their tax burden to smaller local businesses, which sell most of their goods within the state.

For example, in 1998, Michigan adopted what legislators called the single business tax, rewriting state tax law so corporate income tax liabilities are figured on sales only–the single sales factor formula. It was large Michigan manufacturers like Ford Motor Company, with significant property and payroll in state–and few in-state sales–which pushed the act. That same year, Kraft Foods lobbied its home state of Illinois for the same provision. This time, however, Ford Motor opposed Illinois' adoption of the single sales formula, since Ford sells a large number of vehicles in Illinois but has little property or payroll expense there. Three years later, Kraft opposed Maryland's adoption of a similar formula, again because Kraft has little or no property and payroll in the state, but a large amount of sales (CBPP, 2001). Shifting the tax burden away from corporate exporters in Michigan and Illinois had its consequences: By 2003 Illinois had the sixth most regressive tax code in the nation and Michigan the seventh (McIntyre, 2003). Large corporations in these states have shifted their tax bill on to "mom and pop" small businesses. No one knows the total cost of this tax shift; more empirical studies would be useful. There are, however, many specific examples hinting at the overall loss.

When Illinois adopted the single sales formula in 1998, independent analysts calculated the loss to local governments at $63 million annually; the Illinois legislature never released a fiscal note related to the enabling legislation (CBPP, 2001). That $63 million accrued to just five companies, one of which was Motorola (CBPP, 2001). Legislators intended an easing of the tax burden on large in-state manufacturers and hoped to stimulate job growth. By 2001, however, Motorola had closed every manufacturing plant in the state. In fact, between 1998 and 2000, Illinois lost 30,400 manufacturing jobs (CBPP, 2001). This is one of the many examples leading us to question tax policy that has no apparent effect on actual economic development and instead shifts the burden of taxation from large employers to what will become mostly unemployed workers with no ability to pay.

Oregon estimated a 14.8 percent reduction in tax collections should it adopt a single sales factor formula (CBPP, 2001). Instead, policy-makers authored legislation taking effect in May 2003, weighting sales at 80%. Practically speaking, some analysts conclude that once sales factor weighting reaches 70% or greater, property and payroll factors become statistically irrelevant (CBPP, 2001). This change in Oregon's tax structure partially explains the state's budget deficit, which on a biennial basis approached $2 billion in 2003 (CBPP, 2003c), and has not had the desired impact on employment growth. As of August of 2004, only the District of Columbia and Alaska had higher unemployment rates than Oregon's 7.4 percent (BLS, 2004). Fewer financial resources in the state also led to reductions in spending on critical programs.

This type of policy making, according to many observers, represents a zero sum game. Why are lawmakers so willing to amend the tax code when so few benefit, the competitive advantage lasts only in the short term, so little real economic development results, and increasing regressivity threatens the stability and adequacy of government revenues? We find no rational answers to this question. All we can say for sure is, the double-weighted sales factor, and the single sales factor, despite the evidence against them, are the de-facto standards in state tax policy. Table 1 shows the status of state corporate income tax apportionments formulas (as of September, 2004). It is clear that, from a level playing field set by the Multi-State Tax Commission in 1957, many states have moved away from the original equally weighted three factor corporate income tax policy.

THE PASSIVE INVESTMENT CORPORATION

Another lesser-known expenditure results from the *passive investment corporation* (PIC). Under this measure, corporations lease their logos and other intellectual properties from subsidiaries under their control. These subsidiaries typically locate where there is no state cor-

TABLE 1. Status of State Corporate Income Tax Apportionment Formulas

Apportionment formula	States employing them
Three factors, equally weighted	Alabama, Alaska, Delaware, Washington DC, Hawaii, Montana, North Dakota (financial institutions only), Oklahoma, Rhode Island, South Dakota (financial institutions only), Utah, Vermont
Three factors, sales double-weighted	Arizona, Arkansas, California, Connecticut (for manufacturing), Florida, Georgia, Idaho, Indiana, Kentucky, Louisiana, Maine, Maryland, Mississippi (for certain manufacturers and locations, sales only for service and merchandising), New Jersey, New Mexico, New York, North Carolina, South Carolina (for manufacturing), Tennessee, Virginia, West Virginia, Wisconsin
Three factors, sales triple weighted	Ohio, Pennsylvania
Three factors, various weightings	Michigan (90-5-5), Minnesota (75-12.5-12.5), New Hampshire (42.8-28.6-28.6), Oregon (80-10-10)
Two factors only	Kansas (property and sales only), Colorado (revenue and property)
Single sales factor	Illinois, Iowa, Massachusetts (for manufacturers, defense contractors, mutual funds), Missouri, Nebraska, Texas

From data compiled by the Center for Budget and Policy Priorities in: Center for Budget and Policy Priorities. (2001). *The "single sales factor" formula for state corporate taxes.* Washington, DC: Michael Mazerov.

porate income tax. Thus, corporations transfer profits to the subsidiary as payments for use of their intellectual properties. No one explains PICs better than the Center for Budget and Policy Priorities' Michael Mazerov:

> Profits of the operational part of a business that would otherwise be taxable by the state(s) in which the company is located are siphoned out of such states by having the tax-haven subsidiary charge a royalty to the rest of the business for the use of the trademark or patent. The royalty is a deductible expense for the corporation paying it, and so reduces the amount of profit such a corporation has in the states in which it does business and is taxable. Moreover, the "profits" of the PIC are often loaned back to the rest of the corporation, and a secondary siphoning of income occurs through the payment of deductible interest on the loan. (CBPP, 2003a)

Unlike other tax expenditures, where lawmakers have simply failed to calculate the cost and account for them in expenditure budgets, profits transferred into PICs are confidential. States, at times, challenge income tax filings by corporations, and these court cases note the tax payments or revenues in question, giving lawmakers a glimpse into the amount of lost state treasury revenue.

Three examples illustrate what PIC usage costs state governments. The Toys R' Us PIC earned $55 million in 1990 by licensing its name and trademark, among other things, to the parent corporation. That $55 million, like the examples following, escapes any sort of taxation by any state. The PIC affiliated with The Limited group of stores (Victoria's Secret, Lane Bryant, Express) earned $949 million between 1992 and 1994 by licensing trademarks back to the parent stores. Kmart's PIC earned $1.25 billion dollars between 1991 and 1995 using the same method. Other well known companies utilizing PICs as a tax avoidance strategy include Shell Oil, Colgate-Palmolive, Pepsico, Nabisco, General Electric, and Enron–all of whom share or shared a common corporate headquarters in Delaware (CBPP, 2003a).

Delaware and Nevada represent the two most popular states for PIC incorporation since neither state levies corporate income taxes. As of 1998, Delaware boasted 6,000 PICs; one office building in Wilmington hosts 700 "corporate headquarters" on just five floors. Nevada lists 132,000 businesses with no employees, which some analysts say is a reliable indicator that these businesses are PICs. Twenty-two states permit the shifting of corporate income into passive investment corporations (CBPP, 2003a). When quantifying the states with the most regressive tax codes, it is interesting to note that seven out of the top ten most regressive states allow PICs (CBPP, 2003a; McIntyre, 2003).

IS NOWHERE INCOME STILL INCOME?

Nowhere income is income earned by a corporation that escapes taxation by any state, as if the corporation earned it "nowhere." Currently, twenty states allow creation of nowhere income by their resident corporations (CBPP, 2003a), and corporations use two chief methods in creating nowhere income.

The most common strategy exploits differences between state apportionment formulas where one state has a single sales factor formula or some derivative, and others have traditional three-way apportionment formulas. The second strategy is via *remote sales*, typically composed of catalog or Internet sales.

A little known law, *PL 86-272*, allows corporations to avoid paying income tax on profits they earn in states where they have no physical presence. Thirty state tax codes, however, have a *throwback rule* stating that, if a resident company earns profits in a state where there is no tax, the profits are thrown back to the resident state for the purposes of income taxation. The twenty states without the throwback rule allow their resident corporations tax freedom on 50-100% of their profits–nowhere income (CBPP, 2003a). No evidence exists that states, even amidst massive budget shortfalls, are seriously addressing the issue of nowhere income, even though the costs are extraordinary: The Multistate Tax Commission reported in the summer of 2003 that exotic tax sheltering vehicles, such as PICs, the creation of nowhere income, offshore tax havens, and shifting U.S. income to other nations cost states between $8.32 billion and $12.38 billion in corporate income tax revenues (MTC, 2003). Nowhere income is problem enough, but there also exists the issue of how states define traditional business income.

JUST WHAT IS INCOME?

Thirty-nine states define *business income* in a manner that reduces collection of corporate income taxes (CBPP, 2003a). On this subject, there has been virtual legislative inertia. Only two states have made any move whatsoever to tighten their definition of business income, though tax policy literature frequently recommends this change. Little quantitative analysis exists on the issue of defining business income, but where an analysis has been made, it is clear that states are losing significant revenues through ill-constructed corporate tax law. For example, the State of Idaho defines business income as:

> income arising from transactions and activities in the regular course of the taxpayer's trade or business and includes income from the acquisition, management, or disposition of tangible and intangible property when such acquisition, management, or disposition of constitutes integral or necessary parts of the taxpayer's trade or business operations. Gains or losses and dividend and interest income from stock and securities of any foreign or domestic corporation shall be presumed to be income from intangible property, the acquisition, management, or disposition of which constitute an integral part of the taxpayer's trade or business; such presumption may only be overcome by clear and convincing evidence to the contrary. (Idaho Statutes, 2003)

Such a convoluted definition leaves little doubt as to why tax law alienates even fiscal policy stalwarts, let alone most social policy advocates. Professor Walter Hellerstein recommends states simplify the definition of business income to read: "Business income means all income which is apportionable under the Constitution of the United States" (Hellerstein, 2001).

In 2002, the state of North Carolina took Hellerstein's advice, amending its definition of business income in Senate Bill 1115. The Fiscal Research Division of the North Carolina General Assembly estimated that revising their definition of business income would provide the state nearly $290 million, or a 9% increase, in revenues between 2002 and 2007 (Fiscal Division of the North Carolina General Assembly, 2002). Other states could potentially experience the same results, but of the 24 states with non-conforming definitions, only New Jersey followed, prompting one analyst to surmise ignorance and inertia on the part of state legislatures as the prime reason for not amending this law (M. Mazerov, personal communication, November 21, 2003). North Carolina passed this measure with little or no opposition.

PROFITING FROM A NET OPERATING LOSS

Another tax expenditure existing in the shadows is the *net operating loss carry back*. Twenty states allow businesses the option of filing amended tax returns in years where the business makes a profit. A business simply takes current losses, and carries them back to offset the profits made in previous years. This nets all businesses–corporations on down to sole proprietorships–actual cash refunds from state coffers. The flip side of this issue is the net operating loss *carry forward* in which a business carries forward losses from prior years to offset current profits. Economists agree there is some rationale for this sort of income averaging since start-ups typically earn no revenues, but the practice of carry backs is favored only in the ranks of corporate law and accountancy departments. Again, while there is no exact accounting for the total costs of this measure, businesses use it to great advantage. During the depths of the recent economic downturn, (third quarter, 2001) corporate income tax collections fell 32 percent from the same period the year prior; sales, personal income, and corporate income taxes combined fell only 10 percent (CBPP, 2003b).

CONCLUSION

The Center for Public Integrity released a report stating that, ". . . lobbyists and their employers in 39 states spent more than $715 million wining, dining, and generally influencing state lawmakers in 2002" (Center for Public Integrity, 2003) illustrating that lobbyists find particular success with state legislatures and their accompanying treasuries. That $715 million figure excludes the eleven states not reporting lobbying expenditures. The policies that corporate lobbyists, accountants, and lawyers spend hundreds-of-millions of dollars protecting or influencing, are hidden provisions in the tax code, provisions completely unknown to ordinary citizens, and often unknown even to state lawmakers.

Skilled social welfare advocates recognize that legislators increasingly implement social policy via fiscal policy. Too often however, social policy advocates lack the specialized knowledge to confront legislators with poor policy decisions, remaining unable to offer fiscal policy alternatives when advocating for spending on popular social programs. This paper provides insight into some of the more arcane, yet costly, fiscal policies lurking in state tax codes. The social welfare advocate possessing this knowledge can help level the playing field for social welfare programs.

No complete accounting exists for the total loss of revenue to the combined states from tax expenditures. What we do know, however, is that during budget crises, states have responded by increasing regressive taxes and cutting social welfare spending–while leaving costly tax exemptions, deductions, and credits in place. While corporations freely create nowhere income, no state treasury enjoys the corollary: there are no nowhere revenues. As the tax base shrinks and tax policy becomes more regressive, states will find they generate a smaller amount of tax revenue from a decreasing tax base. It will not take an army of economists to predict the outcome. Before those days arrive, states facing budget crises and ever-dwindling treasuries would do well to address the revenue leakages associated with the increased use of state-based tax expenditures.

The job of the social welfare advocate in the face of this reality then, is threefold. First, develop an understanding of intricate fiscal issues by delving more deeply into literature outside of traditional social work journals, for example, fiscal policy analyses done in publications such as *State Tax Notes*, and by groups like the National Association of State Budget Officers, and the Center for Budget and Policy Priorities. Secondly, social policy advocates must learn to communicate in the language of the fiscal experts, and in language the business community and its representatives will both understand and respond to. It is not enough to say that a tax loophole should be closed in the name of "social justice." Social policy advocates may find more success advocating for a loophole closure because it is an outmoded and unsuccessful form of economic development. Lastly, knowing that many existing tax expenditures are regressive, costly, and create little value for the state allows the skilled advocate to create broader and more effective coalitions. Some potential coalition partners are school districts, cities and counties, and small business groups. In any event, it is incumbent upon social welfare advocates to get on the fiscal playing field.

REFERENCES

Arizona Department of Revenue. (2002). *The revenue impact of Arizona's tax expenditures FY 2001/02.* (Arizona Office of Economic Research and Analysis). Phoenix, AZ: Mark W. Killian. Retrieved March 24, 2004, from http://www.revenue.state.az.us/expenditures_2002.pdf

Bader, E., Huff, D., & Reynolds, L. (2003). Shadow welfare: A Cadillac for corporate America. *Social Policy Journal, 2* (4), 39-52.

Brunori, D. (2001). *State tax policy: A political perspective.* Washington, DC: The Urban Institute Press.

Bureau of Labor Statistics. (1999). *Employment and wages annual averages, 1999* (U.S. Department of Labor Bulletin 2534). Washington, DC: U.S. Government Printing Office.

Bureau of Labor Statistics. (2002). *Employment and wages annual averages, 2002* (U.S. Department of Labor). Washington, DC: U.S. Government Printing Office, Retrieved December 16, 2004, from http://www.bls.Gov/cew/ew02sect3133.pdf

Bureau of Labor Statistics. (2004). *Unemployment rates by state, seasonally adjusted, August 2004.* Retrieved December 16, 2004, from http://data.bls.gov/servlet/map.servlet.MapToolServlet?survey=la

Center for Budget and Policy Priorities. (2001). *The "single sales factor" formula for state corporate taxes.* Washington, DC: Michael Mazerov. Retrieved November 21, 2003, from http://www.cbpp.org/3-27-01sfp.pdf

Center for Budget and Policy Priorities. (2002). *States can avoid substantial revenue loss by decoupling from new federal tax provision.* Washington, DC: Nicholas Johnson. Retrieved November 21, 2003, from http://www.cbpp.org/3-20-02sfp.pdf

Center for Budget and Policy Priorities. (2003a). *Closing three common corporate loopholes could raise additional revenues for many states.* Washington, DC: Michael Mazerov. Retrieved November 21, 2003, from http://www.cbpp.org/4-9-02sfp.pdf

Center for Budget and Policy Priorities. (2003b). *Many states could avoid unnecessary revenue loss during the current fiscal crisis by disallowing business operating loss carrybacks.* Washington, DC: Michael Mazerov. Retrieved November 21, 2003, from http://www.cbpp.org/5-20-03sfp.pdf

Center for Budget and Policy Priorities. (2003c). *State budget deficits for fiscal year 2004 are huge and growing.* Washington, DC: Iris J. Lav & Nicholas Johnson. Retrieved November 21, 2003, from http://www.cbpp.org/12-23-02sfp.pdf

Center for Public Integrity. (2003). *Hired guns.* Washington, DC: Robert Morlino, Leah Rush, Derek Willis. Retrieved September 25, 2004, from http://www.publicintegrity.org/hiredguns/report.aspx?aid=165

Evergreen Freedom Foundation. (2004). *Details of Boeing contract.* Retrieved September 21, 2004, from http://www.effwa.org/boeing.php

Fiscal Research Division of the North Carolina General Assembly. (2002). *Legislative fiscal note to Senate Bill 1292.* Raleigh, NC: Fiscal Research Division North Carolina General Assembly. Retrieved November 21, 2003, from http://www.ncga.state.nc.us/ html2001/bills/FiscalInfo/Senate/SFN1292v4.pdf

Flaccus, G. (2003, July 6). Drug problem overwhelms Oregon's Umatilla County. *The Idaho Statesman,* p. A5.

Hancock, J. (1999). S.C. pays dearly for added jobs [Electronic version]. *The Sun News.* Retrieved May 20, 2003, from *http://www.strom.clemson.edu/teams/ced/tax_news/sc-tax-news.html*

Hellerstein, W. (2001, September 3). The business-nonbusiness income distinction and the case for its abolition. *State Tax Notes.*

Idaho Statutes. *Title 63, Revenue and Taxation, Chapter 30, Income Tax-Statute 63-3027 Sec a1.* Boise, ID: State of Idaho. Retrieved September 16, from, http://www3.state.id.us/cgi-bin/newidst?sctid=630300027.K

Institute on Taxation and Economic Policy. (2003). *Who pays? A distributional analysis of the tax systems in all 50 states.* (2nd ed.). Washington, DC: McIntyre, Robert S. et al. Retrieved September 25, 2004, from http://www.itepnet.org/wp2000/text.pdf

Johnston, D. C. (2004). *Perfectly legal.* New York, NY: Portfolio.

Mikesell, J. L. (2001). The tax expenditure concept at the state level: Conflict between fiscal control and sound tax policy. Proceedings from the *National Tax Association's 94th Annual Conference on Taxation.*

Mikesell, J. L. (2003). *Fiscal administration* (6th ed.). Belmont, CA: Wadsworth.

Multistate Tax Commission. (2003). *Corporate tax sheltering and the impact on state corporate income tax revenue collections.* Washington, DC. Retrieved September 12, 2004, from http://www.mtc.gov/TaxShelterRpt.pdf

National Association of State Budget Officers. (2003). *The fiscal survey of states, December 2003.* Washington, DC. Retrieved January 12, 2004, from http://www.nasbo.org/Publications/fiscsurv/fsfall2003.pdf

New Democracy Project. *Closing deficits: Section three–Why business tax revenue is falling behind.* Retrieved November 19, 2003, from http://www.newdemocracyproject.com/publications/closing_deficits/deficits_three.cfm

Oregon Secretary of State. (2004). *Measure 30.* Salem, OR. Retrieved September 21, 2004 from, *http://www.sos.state.or.us/elections/feb032004/guide/m30.htm*

State of Idaho Division of Financial Management. (2003). *General fund revenue book.*

Wallace, J. (2003, December 16). Everett lands 7E7. *Seattle Post Intelligencer.* Retrieved December 16, 2003, from http://seattlepi.nwsource.com/business/152681_boeing16.html?searchpagefrom=1&searchdiff=287

Index

Numbers followed by "f" indicate figures; "t" following a page number indicates tabular material.

BOOK ORDER FORM!

Order a copy of this book with this form or online at:
http://www.haworthpress.com/store/product.asp?sku= 5786

Cutting-Edge Social Policy Research

___ in softbound at $19.95 ISBN-13: 978-0-7890-3206-5 / ISBN-10: 0-7890-3206-6.
___ in hardbound at $39.95 ISBN-13: 978-0-7890-3205-8 / ISBN-10: 0-7890-3205-8.

COST OF BOOKS ________

POSTAGE & HANDLING ________
US: $4.00 for first book & $1.50 for each additional book
Outside US: $5.00 for first book & $2.00 for each additional book.

SUBTOTAL ________

In Canada: add 7% GST. ________

STATE TAX ________
CA, IL, IN, MN, NJ, NY, OH, PA & SD residents please add appropriate local sales tax.

FINAL TOTAL ________
If paying in Canadian funds, convert using the current exchange rate, UNESCO coupons welcome.

❑ **BILL ME LATER:**
Bill-me option is good on US/Canada/Mexico orders only; not good to jobbers, wholesalers, or subscription agencies.

❑ **Signature** ________

❑ **Payment Enclosed: $** ________

❑ **Please charge to my credit card:**

❑ Visa ❑ MasterCard ❑ AmEx ❑ Discover ❑ Diner's Club ❑ Eurocard ❑ JCB

Account # ________

Exp Date ________

Signature ________

(Prices in US dollars and subject to change without notice.)

PLEASE PRINT ALL INFORMATION OR ATTACH YOUR BUSINESS CARD

Name ________

Address ________

City ________ State/Province ________ Zip/Postal Code ________

____

Country ________

Tel ________ Fax ________

May we use your e-mail address for confirmations and other types of information? ❑Yes ❑No We appreciate receiving your e-mail address. Haworth would like to e-mail special discount offers to you, as a preferred customer. **We will never share, rent, or exchange your e-mail address.** We regard such actions as an invasion of your privacy.

Order from your **local bookstore** or directly from
The Haworth Press, Inc. 10 Alice Street, Binghamton, New York 13904-1580 • USA
Call our toll-free number (1-800-429-6784) / Outside US/Canada: (607) 722-5857
Fax: 1-800-895-0582 / Outside US/Canada: (607) 771-0012
E-mail your order to us: orders@haworthpress.com

For orders outside US and Canada, you may wish to order through your local sales representative, distributor, or bookseller.
For information, see http://haworthpress.com/distributors

(Discounts are available for individual orders in US and Canada only, not booksellers/distributors.)

Please photocopy this form for your personal use.
www.HaworthPress.com

BOF06